What Seems To Be The Trouble?

What happens when your health problem just doesn't tick the boxes? One woman's quest for a treatment - any treatment - that would help

Claire Entwistle

ISBN (ebook): 9781234567890

ISBN (paperback): 9798636623731

Cover design by: Creative Covers

Library of Congress Control Number: 2018675309

Printed in the United Kingdom

For Steve, and for Nicola,
and for everyone who has ever tried to help.

Mustn't Grumble

I AM A qualified psychotherapist these days, not a bewildered child, though sometimes I feel like one. I have the right and the means, nowadays, to say whatever I like about illness or disability, though experience suggests that that is no guarantee of being listened to, either by the caring professions or personal loved ones. 'Mustn't grumble', my Northern grandparents used to say when asked about their health. But sometimes I feel like grumbling.

Sometimes I feel like grumbling, and not just about the difficulties of having a health problem, a relatively minor one, God knows, compared to what a lot of people go through, but about the ways in which well-intentioned, highly qualified, free-at-the-point-of-service medical treatment has compounded it. The well-proven cliché in disability circles is that society's attitudes make things hard, not the disability itself. I would add that it is not so very unusual nowadays for medical treatment, and also some of the alternatives, to cause even more problems.

That is what this book is about: based on my own experiences chiefly, because I know them best, and embellished with those of other people I have read about and spoken to. Some of these are inevitably my clients, whose details of course are confidential and not to be mentioned even obliquely, but I cannot help retaining the facts they have told me; and nor would I want to forget.

For me, the trouble was something neurological. Something small. 'A tiny bit of brain damage' hazarded one doctor, when pressed by my twenty-something self. They didn't really know. The same doctor, the first helpful one that I'd met, explained that I was born with a 'small eye' that had stopped developing at some point during gestation. It was covered by a cataract and offered 'no useful vision', as another ophthalmologist put it, accurately, unless you count as useful a faintly red glow when the other eye is covered. The 'good' eye, my left, appeared to be fine at birth, but soon developed a kind of wobble that often goes with neurological problems. The wobble is called nystagmus. I discovered the word at the age of 18, when I got talking to a medical student in freshers week.

Such a shortage of facts. Looking back to my earliest memories, the whole subject remained a blur for much longer than you might expect. I have a theory that in the first shocked months of finding that their second child had a disability, some medic muttered a reassuring 'She'll manage perfectly well', from which my parents concluded that I would behave throughout life exactly as if I had two functioning eyes and a pristine brain. They never referred to the likelihood of any difficulties, even to me, unless it was absolutely necessary. I gradually worked out for myself that something was amiss, and if I managed to phrase a question in the right way, I was rewarded with a straight answer.

'Mummy, did you know that if you cover this eye up with your hand, you can see, but if you cover this one up, you can't?'

'Well, *you* can't, darling. Other people can'.'

'But why…?'

'There's something wrong with you. But don't worry, you'll manage perfectly well.'

Oh. The talk quickly turned to other matters, rather as though I had asked Mum how much money she had in the bank, or what a condom was.

However, the evidence suggests that my parents were talking to somebody about my condition, because when I was four, that person, probably a consultant ophthalmologist, suggested that I should have an operation. I would give a lot to know who that individual was. I expect he (it would be a he, in those days) is dead now. Whoever he was, my parents consented to the surgery, and I was informed.

Memories are fuzzy, but I seem to recall the flavour of the days leading up to the surgery; a pleasant sense of importance, of getting one over on my never-hospitalised big sister. New nighties were purchased, and furry slippers, none of them for her. On the eve of the surgery Mum drove me to the hospital and installed me in my own room with a window overlooking tree tops. There was a crispy bed that went up and down when you pressed a button, and more buttons for when you wanted a drink or to listen to music. Ladies in full-sized nurses uniforms rustled and smiled. It must have been a private ward, but I don't know whether my parents paid or whether it was courtesy of some health insurance. My mother went away as the room grew dark, and in the nightlight's glow, a pale blue nurse gave me Horlicks and tucked me in. Sleep was long in coming, but there came a friendly murmur from the corridor beyond my room, and now and then a kindly face around the door. I seem to remember being happy, that night, as I finally fell asleep.

A plastic cup under my nose. A chemical stench. 'Drink it. No, drink all of it'. My throat fighting the terrifying bitterness, struggling and failing to vomit. 'Finish it all'. A hand clenching the back of my head. It must have been the pre-med, administered by mouth as a kinder alternative to a needle. Turns out that there are worse things than needles.

Swimming upwards from black to black. Trying and failing to scream. Something in my throat. My throat sliced vertically down the middle, its two halves glued together, no room to breathe.

'You want water?'

'Yes.'

'To swill your mouth out, or swallow?'

'Swallow.'

'Then you can't have it.' Down to the deeper darkness.

I don't know if that conversation really happened. I remember the long hours after waking up properly and finally, finally, feeling the lap of lukewarm liquid on my furrowed tongue. Then I remember the ripping off of bandages, the prodding at my fugitive eye with sticks and spikes, the agonising daylight, injunctions to wrench apart my own lids to count held-up fingers that merged and waved. This nightmare repeated itself, perhaps daily, perhaps more. Sometimes my parents were there, or the nurses, sometimes not; I didn't really care. I cared for cool drinks, and stillness, and the echo of an empty floor; the distancing of the enemy.

Eventually the bandages came off permanently and I was allowed to go home. There followed check-ups, first at the hospital and then the local optician's, more finger counting, and much adulation for the perpetrator of these horrors.

'Here, look at those stitches! A textbook job.'

This invitation to admire my surgeon's dexterity would be addressed by the optician to white-coated colleagues or passing students, not to me, which was fortunate because only my clenched teeth and pursed lips were holding back a scream of colossal proportions, possibly the same scream that failed to make it through my desiccated windpipe on the day of the surgery. Oh, the pain and terror of that little red beam – to this day, I quail before a bright light in the darkness – the icy advance of those metal instruments.

These follow-up appointments, at intervals of weeks then months, meant a morning off school followed by my favourite lunch of kippers and meringues. Bizarrely I always looked forward to that lunch, as if I couldn't retain a sense of the awfulness of the procedures themselves. If this sounds muddled, that is because it was. It was as if part of me refused to believe what was happening, even as another part howled and raged. I know now that this 'splitting' is common in cases of trauma, and also that 'trauma' is the correct term for certain medical experiences, from dental work to childbirth.

'Oh well', I seem to hear some optimistic soul remark, 'there we go, nobody much enjoys seeing the optician, any more than the dentist, but the operation was worth it because you could see better afterwards, right?'

Wrong, but it took me years to find out why. The operation was never intended to help me see better, exactly. It was the same operation that is given to children who squint, tightening up the muscles around the eye. People with nystagmus often have what is called a 'null point', a position where the involuntary movement reduces and their sight improves. So they tend to instinctively adopt a head position which puts their steadiest vision directly in front of them. My null point was over to the left, and the head posture started in my earliest months. The baby photos in the family album depict a robust but lopsided infant, her beaming face turning to the right.

'OK', nods my protagonist, 'So the operation was successful in a different way, and it made you see straight in front without twisting your head, right?'

Wrong again. The stitches remained text-book neat, but their effect wore off after a few months, and my head posture was exactly the same as before. You can see it in the nursery school photos: a pale and wary waif, with a head tilt to the right.

'Oh. So the doctors recognised that the surgery hadn't worked and regretted all that wasted stress, did they?'

No regrets, no, but they did offer to do it again... they *recommended* doing it again!

'But still, your parents realised what the surgery had been like the first time, and refused, right?'

Well, no. I don't recall ever telling them what it had been like for me, or being asked. Perhaps I assumed that they realised, and that recurrent butchery was inevitable, like having my hair washed. When my mother informed me, aged six, that I would be going back into hospital during the spring half term, I just accepted it, packing my own bag this time. I don't recall being particularly worried. Perhaps, I suspect now with hindsight, I went a bit blank. Trauma does that.

'So did the results last better the second time?'

Nope. The family holiday photos from that summer show a red and angry child, hugging a book in the dimmest corner of the beach, with a head tilt to the right.

What seems to be the trouble?

THAT IS WHAT doctors say by way of an introduction, here in the UK, or they did when I still used to speak to them. What *seems* to be the trouble? Establishing at the start that whatever you the patient have to say about your experience may prove illusory; the doctor will be the one to say what actually *is* the trouble.

'Come, come', says the hypothetical cheery chappy who took it for granted that operations on small children do more good than harm, and maintains his position against the evidence of my family album. 'Come, come, that's a bit sweeping. Doctors listen to how you're feeling, then they give you the benefit of their experience.'

Hmm. He needs a name, this character whose experience has been so far from mine that we might be speaking different languages. Rodney, that will do. Rodney is someone whose experience of conventional medicine is uniformly positive. His broken leg was set in hospital and treated by a lovely physio called Louise until he regained his former brisk walk. His mother had breast cancer ten years ago, but she's out of danger now. He's thankful that his sons are immunised against the child-killers of not so long ago. And all for free! He loves the NHS, does Rodney, and won't hear a word against it.

Rodney does not live in my world.

Neither did that surgeon who decided to operate a second time without thinking to check what it had been like for me. How would that dialogue with my parents have gone?

'It can happen that the head posture returns after a first operation, but there's a seventy per cent chance that repeat surgery will reduce the head tilt by fifty to ninety per cent, for an average sixteen and a half years'.

Those figures are my own, drawn out of the air.

And my parents would have replied:

'Well, that's a pretty good success rate, and the insurance covers it, so why not? Give the dear girl another chance. She does look a bit odd with her head lolling around.'

I believe that they meant well, but it would have been nice if they'd thought to ask whether I wanted to go through that again. What were they thinking of? They are both dead now, like the original set of doctors (probably), so I can't ask either of them.

I digress. What did seem to be the trouble, at this stage of my life, going through primary and then secondary school? I was nervous, not so much of people but in a very physical way: shocked by sudden movements, especially near my face; tending to scream if my scarf blew up in the breeze or an insect brushed my cheek. My sense of balance was terrible. I sank to the ground with ridiculous frequency, like a felled tree, when attempting to walk on uneven ground or looking over the mildest of precipices. I was frequently sick and dizzy, and subject to throat and breathing problems.

My neck hurt most of the time, my head was too heavy and I was always looking for things to rest it on. I had terrible nightmares about knives and kidnapping. If the light was turned on in my bedroom on a dark winter's morning, I screamed and covered my face.

As if all this was not bad enough, I was sure that the house we lived in was haunted, though come to think of it other people had the same opinion, so it may not have been a symptom of post-surgery trauma. This is the difficulty in saying what the trouble really was. It troubled me to think that the house was haunted, but quite likely there were other explanations for the extreme cold in the dining room, the static crackling of the air, the sense of dread where the old staircase used to stand. There could have been other explanations for all that nausea and nerviness and hyper-arousal, as I would call it now. There is no way that I can remember clearly how light-sensitive or wobbly I was before the age of four; I might have been just as bad pre-surgery.

How can we ever know? There would have to be a controlled trial: another Me, born into the same family at the same time, with the same neurological condition, but no operations. If funding were available, there would be a third Me, with conditions the same, but no disability or illness. Then I'd know. Then I could tell those doctors, and perhaps even convince Rodney, that harm had been done to me, terrible, lasting harm, not a temporary discomfort.

'Harm, from the NHS? Do you have any idea how lucky you are?'

Oh, Rodney! Would I be more credible if I first established that Bupa paid for that surgery, and that I am not, in any way, dissing the NHS? I'm grateful for the NHS, really I am. I'm grateful to know that if I ever get hit by a car – which is not unlikely, with cars approaching from the right at a pace beyond my visual capacities, and especially with the advent of silent-assassin electric vehicles – if or when I get hit by a car, an ambulance will arrive and painkillers will make me comfortable and surgeons will sew me together and antibiotics will keep the sepsis away. I'm deeply grateful to the brave souls putting in ungodly hours of messy, demanding, traumatic work, especially those receiving little pay. Thank God, thank God for them: I do not begrudge a penny of my National Insurance payments. What I am saying here – Rodney, are you listening? - is that modern medicine does not work for everyone all the time, and that sometimes it does harm. A lot of harm. And harm is the last thing doctors are meant to do. What happened to the Hippocratic Oath?

Rodney, who is a nice man really, a homely man who has his own children and cares about education, is more interested in how I managed at school with the visual impairment side of things. Oh, that. Fine, most of the time. The vision in my left eye was pretty good; still is. No problems with writing or reading anything that I could hold close enough. I flourished in subjects like English and French, even Latin, which involved more books than blackboards. Focusing on the board, even from the front row, was such hard work that my eyes swam and ached after a few seconds, so I fell behind in chalk-based activities, maths being the worst. And games: I was absolutely incompetent at tennis and hockey. My involuntary eye movement plus the lack of binocular vision made a fast-moving ball disappear when it left the protagonist's hand, sometimes reappearing with a thud between my eyes, with predictable results on the screaming front. Eventually I was let off games, largely

I suspect for the benefit of my peers, who didn't want me on their team.

Socially, it was not too bad at school. The small classes in the small schools I attended suited me, keeping things close. Further afield, objects and people didn't appear blurred so much as lacking in detail; I could see quite clearly a person standing a few yards away, but not what their face looked like. I made a few friends and don't remember ever being bullied, though being bad at sport made for routine rejections. Teachers on the whole were sympathetic, kind even, but not in any practical way. My geography teacher won the award for the most accurate and least constructive remark, when she wrote on my school report, next to the 16% I had achieved in the mock O Level: 'Claire did badly this year because she could not see the board'. I was let off taking the O Level itself, largely I suspect for the benefit of the school's statistics.

Rodney is reassured. All fine there, then. My parents thought the same, I suppose. We didn't ever discuss it. I passed enough exams to get into university at a time when only one in ten 18-year-olds went. And after re-enacting the school blackboard problems at the university whiteboard, I got a degree! And then I got a job! Success all round!

The top ten per cent? Straight into graduate work? No trouble there, then. But there was trouble, it seemed to me. The nausea was troubling, and the dizziness, and the quite spectacular motion sickness, which if anything increased with age. ('Haven't you grown out of it yet?' my aunt would ask every time she saw me. Childless herself, she liked the idea of taking her nieces for lovely drives, pointing out fast-moving objects of interest along the twisting country lanes. She's dead now too.)

And the light sensitivity! My God. The agony of facing a sunny window, or worse, sitting in a vehicle with passing trees flick-flick-flicking the glare into my left eye. It was always my left eye in a car, even as an adult, because I was always the passenger, being unable to drive myself, or to sit in the back without feeling even worse.

'So, what seems to be the trouble today?'

The doctor is annoyed because I've arrived late, by about ten seconds. I misread the room number on the electronic sign in the waiting room – 'B', not '8' – and had to run back to check at reception. He is seated at his computer, and the chair for the patient is positioned against the short side of the desk, so that he is out of sight unless I twist my head all the way round to the right. Ouch. Should I move the chair a little? No, he didn't like it when it did that last time. Or was that another doctor? I have assumed the present tense because this scenario played itself out so often that the instances merge together.

'My neck really hurts. Here, and here and here.'

He prods where I point, and I wince.

'That's just muscular. Nothing to worry about. I'll give you a prescription for painkillers if you like, but you can get them cheaper at Boots. Everything else alright?'.

'I don't really want to take painkillers, because they make me feel sick. I feel sick most the time anyway. And dizzy. It's really bad, some days I just keep falling over.'

'Most of the time? You may have an ear infection.'

A pause while he shoves his freezing torch into my ears. I cringe as it approaches my face.

'There's no sign of infection, but there isn't always. We can try penicillin, just in case.'

This particular memory must be from before they started

cutting down on antibiotics. But at that time, would there have been an electronic sign in reception? I can recall the outline of these appointments, not the detail.

'Um – I'd rather not, unless it is definitely an infection.'

I was ahead of my time on that one, partly because antibiotics had made me horribly sick in the past, and partly because pills of any kind made my gorge rise. That would be part of the controlled trial: would the non-operated-on Me have a problem with swallowing drugs? Would the Me without the neurological issues experience fewer side effects?

The doctor's fingers, drumming his desk just beyond my field of vision, suggest that my eight minutes are up and that as patients go I am deeply unsatisfactory. A young woman shouldn't be coming back year after year with these vague symptoms which he associates with the menopausal sad, and not even having the courtesy to take what is offered.

And after all, I muse, as I thank him and leave the room, what was I expecting? Doctors prescribe drugs. Drugs and surgery. I should know that, if anyone does. Repeat prescriptions, repeat dialogue. The doctors as interchangeable as their consulting rooms: male pattern baldness above weary eyes, a narrow couch opposite a wooden desk, the chairs always orientated to extort the maximum right head-turn from the patient.

Rodney, who has been worrying about his own hairline and wondering what the NHS can do, sighs a bit. He really can't see what all the fuss is about.

Yes, But

I WAS IN my early twenties when I first considered seeking help outside conventional medicine.

I was no longer living at home at this time. I moved out the day following my return from university. I had warned my parents on the phone that I would be doing this, but they either hadn't listened or hadn't believed me, because there was an awkward moment when I mentioned my plan face to face. We were drinking a welcome home Martini on the dining room window seat, one of the more sinister areas of the house, but bearable in daylight and in company.

I accepted a drink from Dad, raised my glass to theirs and extracted my sandalled foot from a current of icy air that snaked in from the balmy, blue-skied garden. My foot was still freezing; I tucked it under my skirt and did up my cardigan. Foiled.

'Could I have a lift to the station in the morning, because I'm starting the job on Monday and I'd like to settle into the new flat? Oh, cheers.'

'But darling!' Mum put down her glass and placed her hand on mine. 'You said the job is near Waterloo. You could be there in an hour, door to door. Why not stay at home?'

The faintest outline of a grinning face seemed to form

against a panelled recess behind her head. I spilt my drink, groped for tissues and looked again. Nothing there.

'Thanks, but no. I'm grown up now. I should be independent.'

Dad shook his head.

'You could live here and be independent!'

But neither of them could put up a convincing case for my remaining, having made it clear many times that once I reached majority, they would consider their job done. I had been a bit shocked the first time I was informed of this, aged twelve, but I was used to the idea now, and surprised that they seemed less than ready to follow through.

Much later, a counsellor suggested that I left home so promptly not because the house was haunted or because I'd learnt to value independence, but because I was angry with my parents.

'*No! Why on earth would I be?*'

'Because they made you have those operations?'

It had never occurred to me; we always got on fine, and I was fond of Mum especially; but now the counsellor mentioned it… Yes, you can go off people. I certainly, from my earliest years, did not trust either of them a single inch.

Rodney doesn't like me saying that. He does the best for his boys and is sure that other parents do likewise. I'm not saying that they meant any harm, Rodney, I'm saying that they weren't careful enough. Like the system which decided on those operations and carried them out. Yes, I was angry. I'm angry now.

So I moved into a run-down South London flat-share with an articled clerk and two nurses, and begin to enjoy the independence with which I had been threatened since pre-teen years. Away from the pressures of university and the sinister whiff of home, I felt light and free. It wasn't ideal living with medical folk, hearing stories of life on the wards and shuddering at the early-morning rustle of uniforms when the girls were on nights, but as soon as they were back in their jeans, we laughed together a lot – at the black-and-white television whose sound failed so regularly that we had to ad-lib our own dialogue; at our other flatmate's messy attempts to smoke a pipe; at our landlord's insistence that the flat was a prestigious place, despite his repeated visits to disguise with emulsion paint the front bedroom's human-sized damp patch, which we christened Desmond.

My first job was a short-term fundraising contract for a charity which involved giving talks all around the country, persuading students to sign up for a standing order. I enjoyed giving the talks, and was rather successful at signing people up, but my neurological condition put a minor kibosh on the pleasure in it. It was hard work galloping through the rush hour to mainline stations, craning my neck at information boards, wandering around strange campuses in search of charity reps whom I failed to re-identify once they had walked away for a moment. The days were long – I went to Aberystwyth once to give a ten minute talk – and some nights I got home too dizzy and disorientated even to watch the telly.

I had never imagined wanting to work in an office, but I began to crave repetitious journeys to work, free evenings and an identifiable set of colleagues. A friend suggested I fill in a form for the civil service – that sounded static enough – and they offered the option of learning computer programming in a building within walking distance of the flat. This prospect was so pleasing that I chose to ignore the implications of all that close work on screens and coding sheets (this was back in the 80s). The lifelong 'yes, but' aspect of finding a job which suited my capacities, was underway. Yes, giving talks sounded manageable, but there was all the travel and the coping with unfamiliar places. Yes, an office job would be easier to negotiate, but there was the close work to deal with. This was after eliminating all the jobs where a driving licence was required, and those where anybody with a disability was automatically excluded, as vocations such as nursing and teaching were in those days, in practice if not in theory.

My parents, whom I phoned weekly and visited monthly, were pleased that I'd found a steady job, and I find it surprising now that they did not mention any concern that the constant staring at screens might be problematic. They clearly retained their first faith in that specialist who claimed, possibly as a throwaway comment, that I'd manage perfectly well with one eye. Perhaps if Mum and Dad had voiced this expectation in so many words, I would have contested it, but their silent injunction to just get on with it was more insidious and more powerful than any number of words.

So I accepted the IT job in the civil service, on the fifth floor of a high-rise block in the middle of the Elephant and Castle roundabout, under a sign which some joker had vandalised to read 'Alexander lemming House'. I started on 18 December and for the first fortnight had sole occupation of the office. My line manager had left me a book called 'How To Code' and a note that he'd be back in the new year. Rather a minimalist introduction to my new career, but I didn't mind. I enjoyed sitting in a warm room above the buzz of the Elephant and Castle traffic, drinking Nescafé and working through the 'How To Code' book. It was like maths without the blackboard.

In January my two room-mates arrived: Tim, who was

single and treated the office like a home from home, storing his collection of biking magazines in the filing cabinets and ordering takeaway pizza when he had flexi-time to catch up, and Phil, who was married and phoned his wife twice a day, at lunchtime to check how her day was going and at home time to see what shopping she needed. Tim at twenty-six was allegedly still a virgin, at least according to Phil, who showed much interest in the matter. Phil's own conjugal duties, their permutations and locations, were endlessly speculated on by Tim. Our three desks were pushed together, my colleagues facing each other and I between them.

I said as little as possible about my life, especially in relation to the boyfriend I had recently acquired via my flat mates, but my reticence only provided greater scope for their imaginings. Closing my ears to their chatter, I bent over my coding sheets and, when my turn came round, pressed my nose to the monitor we shared. There was no doubt that it was visually tiring, and I made a lot of mistakes, mostly to do with transposing numbers and missing out lines. I was deeply nervous of exposure during the first months, but in fact the management were pleased with me. 'You are the only one in that room doing any work,' confided the Senior Principal during payday night drinks, leaving me shocked that doing some work – any work – was so unusual as to invite comment.

I loved being paid; it made me feel responsible and safe, emphasising my non dependence on my parents. Things were easier in those days for young graduates, and my London salary more than covered my room and other necessities. My boyfriend was an earnest young activist who gave most of his own money to charity and insisted on the cheapest of dates – half a pint in our local, or a Marmite sandwich at a free concert. He also deplored the purchase of any new clothing, preferring, when his own leather belt broke, to replace it with a luggage strap. Thus our social life required only minimal outlay on my part too, and I had money put by for luxuries.

What luxuries did I yearn for? Oh, for pearls beyond price – a pain-free neck, a clear head, a sweet dream, a nausea-free car ride. The desk job which I had hoped would reduce my stress was leaving me shattered and shaky by the evening. I resorted to registering with my local GP and went to see him complaining – ha! another significant word; patients' reports of their symptoms are 'complaints' rather than 'descriptions' -- complaining of severe head and neck pain that drilled right into my jaw. The doctor did all the usual 'Just muscular', 'Could be a virus' banter, then added 'Being a civil servant would make anyone's jaw ache'.

This remark cheered me up a bit, unlike the prescription, whose effects were depressingly familiar. It came with a closely-printed leaflet listing as side effects most of the symptoms I was taking it for (headache, nausea, dizziness, even nystagmus), and it introduced me to the phenomenon that it is possible to feel dizzy on more than one plane, as it were, at a time. I also developed the chills and the dry mouth advertised on the leaflet. I tried to be grateful that I had avoided the constipation and, better still, the renal failure.

You can go off people, and you can go off conventional medicine too. After three days of swallowing this torture in pill form I woke early with a parched mouth to the rubber soles of the nurses creeping up the stairs, and decided in that moment that enough was enough. There must be another way, an alternative – an alternative treatment – and I was going to find it.

Rodney put his head round the door and said he thought I was making a grave mistake. I threw my pillow at him.

Back In The Room

I HAD NO idea where to look for an alternative treatment, with Google far in the future and the whole complementary medicine industry yet to take off, and most of my acquaintances contented Rodneys who would have suggested asking my GP for a second opinion or a different drug.

I asked my boyfriend what he would do in my place, but he could only suggest sending the money to Nicaragua. I looked up into his pale face – he was very tall – and wondered what on earth I was doing with someone with whom I had so little common understanding. Come to think of it, I had started going out with him in the first place mostly because he seemed to expect that I would. We'd both been invited to a very crowded party, and I'd sat down next to him, failing to wonder why this was the only free chair in the room, and said hello. He was almost speechless at the time, but at the end of the evening he told me to meet him in the local pub the following night, and I did.

We had some things in common, obviously. We had what are nowadays called shared values, up to a point; I too worried about poverty and homelessness and political instability; but unlike him, I wasn't willing to set aside my own well-being to right these wrongs. I still found him attractive, and could see that he had many excellent qualities, but you can go off people, and I went off him at the moment when he said, in effect, that it didn't matter how bad I felt. We stopped seeing each other from that day, without any great drama, and perhaps this leant an air of even greater unreality to the next few weeks. I didn't try asking anyone else I knew their opinion of alternative therapies. I didn't want to overturn my flatmates' idea of me as a mostly healthy person, and I suspected my other friends might have thought me weird. The thought of consulting my parents never occurred.

In the end I tried the local library, and after a few evenings browsing the personal development section and local newspapers, decided on hypnotherapy. 'Feel less pain… sleep better… experience a new confidence and freedom'. Apparently the practitioner sat some distance from the patient, and no foreign objects were introduced or bodily fluids exchanged, yet the brain – the seat and origin of all my problems – would be soothed, coaxed, gentled to a happier state. What could possibly go wrong?

I soon found out.

The hypnotherapist I chose was a woman called Annie who worked from her home in Docklands, an easy journey from where I lived. It took a couple of phone calls to find a time we could both make; she only seemed to have one or two appointments free each week, always around noon, which meant I had to arrange a whole day's annual leave. But it seemed a good sign that she was so sought-after, and the wait gave me time to enjoy the sense of impending change, impending healing, impending new life. I felt better already!

On the day of my appointment I woke up feeling fine – excited, hopeful, not dizzy, not sick. I cheerily negotiated the path from the tube station, strolled along the banks of a strangely tidy canal, and arrived ten minutes early at the door of her new-build terrace. That was when my confidence started to go. I stood staring at her door, a thick slab of uPVC punctured with highly-polished smoked-glass panels which didn't look at all like a gateway to peace and healing. Eventually I rang the bell to find that Annie, throwing wide the portcullis, was highly-polished herself, with Teflon hair and a silky black suit. She smiled, sort of, and hurried me in.

'Leave your shoes there.'

I struggled with laces, aligned my trainers with her leather boots, and followed her heels into a cream and wood living room. Those shoes! She might have been on her break from some city firm! Come to think of it, she had only offered appointments around lunchtime. I was scared now, the more so when she pointed to a couch under a sun-dazzled window. I edged on to it and closed my eyes.

Daylight blazed in. My eyelids, tissue-thin, sizzled.

'Can we...,' I cleared my throat, 'Can we close the blinds?'

Annie frowned.

'No! I need light. I need to read your expression. Just relax.'

Suddenly I was a child back in hospital. The poisoned chalice of pre-med thickened in my throat. I sat up and shielded my eyes.

'I can't relax like this.'

'You'll be fine. You'll relax in no time.'

She started to talk, leading me down a wide staircase towards a dim landing. That would have suited me fine, but my eyelids reported no reduction in glare. I cannot imagine what my expression looked like, that she was so carefully monitoring: my eyes scrunched up, my pulse thumping, my teeth clenched. But I persevered, counting down the stairs, 7,8,9 until we reached the bottom and I was invited to approach a large book that lay on an oak table.

Annoyingly, I did actually see the book and, as instructed, began to turn the pages backwards. The font was tiny and cramped, as if composed by a pedantic lawyer. It was only when we reached the back cover and I was invited to keep turning imaginary pages, that I realised the woman was a past-life regression therapist. No! Oh, no! This current life was more than enough to cope with. I glimpsed shadows, the form of that face that appeared in the panelled dining room at home. Oh, no, no! I wrenched the page the other way, filtering out Annie's drone, and stared at a sheet of painful white until it was time to go back up the stairs. 3,2,1, you're back in the room.

I sat up and glared. Annie stroked a strand of raven hair, smiling sleepily. She looked completely different from the bossy power-dresser who had sneered at my trainers. Hypnotism clearly calmed and rejuvenated her, as claimed in her advert.

'My dear, you went very deep. What did you see?'

'Nothing. A blank sheet.'

Inky lashes dipped and rose.

'You are deeply relaxed. You will sleep well tonight. You may find that your dreams tell you more.'

She looked at her watch. Ten to two. Perhaps she was due back at the day job for a 2pm meeting. I scrambled into my shoes, stumbled outside and leant against a wall, gasping with helpless longing. I had really hoped, believed almost, that something might… Behind me, Annie left the house and hurried towards the office blocks.

That cost me £60. It was a lot of money in those days.

'Oh well', says Rodney, giving his own chin a sympathetic rub. 'You gave it a go. You left it there, right?'

Wrong.

How You Say?

AT THE TIME I felt guilty and silly, seeking out a similar experience straight after this disaster, but from my current perspective as an experienced psychotherapist it seems 'healthy', as we therapists say, that I didn't give up on alternative treatments on the basis of one bad experience with Annie. Bad, but not really as bad as all that. It was disappointing that Annie didn't take seriously my request for a dimmer environment, but not her fault that I lacked, at that time, the mental welly to insist on it. It was certainly not her fault that I didn't think to check what kind of hypnotherapist she was, because her past-life proclivities cannot have been secret.

And was Annie really as inexperienced as I feared? The younger Me has laid out evidence that Annie was moonlighting from a job in the City in order to get my reader onside in doubting her expertise, but I know now that therapists have to pay for their training somehow, and that they don't achieve a full practice immediately after qualifying. More importantly, Annie didn't do me any actual harm, and in fact I did sleep well that night, exhausted by the emotion of it all and missing, for the first time, my boyfriend, whom I had somehow managed to forget about immediately after finishing with him. So in retrospect it doesn't seem such a bad thing that I took a breath then started looking about for an alternative alternative therapist who might suit me better.

The somebody I thought might suit me better was a very small, very young-looking, very quietly-spoken man called Yin who rented a room above a local health-food store which sold a particular brand of dried olives that were an acceptable substitute for the peppermints I was always trying to give up. I used to mindlessly reread his leaflets whilst queuing at the till, and I even caught a glimpse of him once. He was helping an elderly patient upstairs, relieving her of her bag and telling her to take her time. Frankly, Annie had been a bit terrifying, and I had no notion at this stage of women being any safer than men, and Yin's leaflet showed that he offered in addition to hypnotherapy something called EMDR, which dealt with rapid eye movements. That sounded extremely relevant to me. Yin was my man, and I booked an appointment.

'… and I get startled easily, and dizzy, and I have bad dreams, and I'd like something to calm it all down.'

In the upstairs room, Yin scribbled a couple of notes, then leant across his desk.

'Very good. Let me tell you about EMDR'.

I was sitting straight across from him, which was good, but it was disconcerting to see this doctor-style desk and beyond it a narrow couch. And why was there so little light in the room? Was that a net curtain, or a blind? My inability to make out detail was infuriating sometimes. I squinted and put my head further to the side, angling for a better view. Not that I wanted the beastly sun glaring in, but a bit of natural light would cheer things up. I was starting to feel quite depressed, even anxious. And how come I had missed what Yin was saying?

'... so that is how it works. In short, EMDR moves the memory of your bad experience from one part of the brain to another part which can deal with it better'.

'OK. So what happens next?'

'You recall a memory of the matter that is causing you distress.'

I was flummoxed. 'There isn't anything really. My joints hurt. I wake up in the night, screaming.'

Yin did not even nod. Hello? Had I perhaps not spoken?

'There is no need to describe me the memory, just to recall it, and to hold it in your mind, with the feelings it arouses.'

A pulse started beating in my throat. I felt hot.

'But there isn't anything.'

'You must search your mind. You will find it.'

I searched my mind. Ah - whenever I woke after a nightmare, I felt panicky about the knives, or the ghosts, or whatever it was. I summoned up the flush of those moments, the pounding heart.

'OK, I've got something.'

Yin came round the desk and stood over me. He thrust his right hand towards my face, and began to flick it backwards and forwards right in front of my eyes. I gasped. I pressed back into my chair and screwed up my eyelids.

'Open your eyes. Pay attention.' Was this the man who took the elbow of that frail lady?

I opened my eyes and after a moment of fumbling (these things are harder with monocular vision), I seized his moving hand in my fist, shoving it into his chest. We stared at each other, both breathing fast. I recovered first.

'Sorry. I'm… not good with things near my face. I should have told you. My fault.'

He nodded and retreated round the desk.

The clock on his wall showed only fifteen minutes gone, and I had paid in advance for an hour and a half. The sixty pounds I wasted on Annie still rankled. I must not storm out, or worse, do anything to make him chuck me out.

'So sorry. Did I say I wanted EMDR? Silly of me. I meant hydrotherapy. No, hypnotherapy!'

Yin looked doubtful.

'What for?'

'I get a bit nervous sometimes.' We both looked at my hands, clasped on my side of the table. They were shaking, almost bouncing off the wooden surface.

Yin nodded slowly.

'All right then. We can work on giving you more confidence in yourself. You seem vulnerable. You need protection.'

Protection sounded good. I lay down on the couch in the blessed dimness from what revealed itself, when approached, as a linen blind. There was a leather chair beside the couch which Yin pulled back a few feet before sitting down, possibly at what he considered a safe distance.

It was nice to be lying flat. The stabbing in my left hip and the ache in my right shoulder, both of which had been severe for the last few days, calmed themselves. I asked for, and was given, a blanket.

'You are standing at the top of a long flight of steps…'

Down those stairs again, and perhaps it was easier having done the same thing chez Annie. I really did 'relax more at every step'.

'And now,' floated Yin's voice from a long, long way

away, 'And now, you step into a hall, a beautiful hall with beautiful panelling on the walls, and you see a long oak table, and laid on the table is a suit of armour.'

And there it was.

'There is a breastplate. Do you see it?'

'Mmm'.

'Pick it up, and put it on.'

It was the spitting image of some armour we had seen in a museum on a primacy school trip, and had been allowed to touch; it had felt like lead, and our little hands could barely raise it. This breastplate in the panelled hall, when heaved over my head, had straps that dug into my neck muscles and sent my head wobbling.

'Now the leg plates.' My hip stabbed in alarm.

'And the helmet.' Ouch! Poor head, already so heavy.

A few minutes later it seemed that I was trotting around on a horse, taking a pop at my adversaries with some kind of rifle. The sight of guns had upset me ever since I saw my dad shoot a squirrel, and the single horse-riding lesson I attempted represented my most terrifying and humiliating experience of sport. A memory resurfaced of clambering atop a snorting monster and sliding, head-first, off the other side. At this point, Yin may have noticed that all was not well, because he varied the script, and the horse and the armour, thank God, melted away.

'You are at your school sports day, and you are doing so well. You are coming first in every single race and winning every single game'.

I could only see myself coming last in every single race. No amount of staircases could remove the hard-wiring in my brain: sports day, with its bossy adults pointing at things I could not make out, and its excitable children making unpredictable movements, and its rows of staring faces, was an unmitigatedly bad thing. But what did Yin know of my inner world, its terrors and humiliations? He could only speak for himself: as an athlete, a rider, a lover of tales of derring-do.

Eventually I was allowed back up the stairs, and I thanked Yin for his help, declined to make another appointment just now, and walked alone down the literal staircase, my hand trembling on the bannister.

Rodney is laughing, he can't help it. I'm laughing, too. It really is funny, in its way, that If Yin had studied my background and psychology for months, he could not have devised redder rags for my internal bull.

'Anyway,' says Rodney, blowing his nose and wondering if he's getting a cold, 'You gave up after that, right?'

Well, no! Reflecting on this fact, I begin to sympathise with the 'Surely this time will be different' position which led to me having two failed eye operations. EMDR was out of the question for obvious reasons, but the very ghastliness of my first two hypnotherapy experiences made me think that if only the 'script' was angled to meet my needs, it might help a lot. I was obviously quite suggestible; I had found it only too easy to conjure up the sinister 'book of my life', the prancing warhorse and the childhood sports field.

Also I suspected what seems crystal clear now: that the intensity of my response to flickering lights and motion was not entirely neurological, but partly habit. Mum used to complain that as a small child, I would throw up as soon as I got into a coach; the sight, sound and smell of the vehicle being enough to set off my motion sickness. Maybe hypnotherapy, by suggesting a different way of thinking about travel, could break that habit.

So it happened that a few months later, I started looking for a different kind of hypnotherapist, one with the crucial missing quality: a recognition that the 'script' had to be right for the client. And I found somebody who seemed to fit this bill. Lucy, her name was — a simple, non-threatening name if ever there was one. Her leaflet stipulated that potential clients had to fill in a form before booking a session, explaining what their problem was and suggesting an image that might be used to resolve it. Lucy would then decide, before any money changed hands, whether this was something she could work with.

I fell on this fascinating task. After several drafts, I focused on travel sickness as my central problem, especially the flick-flick-flick of the light coming into my eyes from the left. My chosen visualisation involved turning the light into little arrows which softened as they approached my face, so that they fell gently to the ground without touching me, without even disturbing me. I practised this a few times on my own, morphing flickering lights into dripping honey. Then I visualised getting into a car on a sunny day, and I certainly felt less apprehensive than usual. I knew it — I was a good hypnotherapy subject! I wondered for a moment whether I needed a professional at all.

Lucy rang up as soon as she received my form, sounding rather impressed by the thoroughness of my response, and I went to see her in her office above a dry cleaners. She was younger than I'd expected, and more eager, leaning forward in her chair and sweeping golden curls back from her heart-shaped face, her voice a-tremble with enthusiasm. She had sounded experienced in her leaflet, but I started to fear that like Annie she spent most of her time on other work, perhaps even downstairs, wrapping chemical-scented clothes in cellophane. But I was committed now, and lay down quickly before my nerve could fail. Lucy introduced the inevitable staircase, I trudged downstairs for the third time, and out came the arrows.

'The arrows are coming, sharp little metal arrows, they're coming towards your head; they're going into your eyes, through your eyes, and when they reach your brain, they start to melt in the heat...' Oh God! She'd put red-hot bloody metal right inside my brain. I pressed my fists into my eyes and managed not to scream. Enough! No more Miss Compliant Client. I sat up. I sat up, in the middle of a hypnotherapy session! I got right off the couch and told her, as politely as was manageable, that this was not what I had meant. Wrong sort of arrows!

'Oh,' said Lucy, lining up her ballet pumps and looking very meek and very sweet, and very unlike the kind of professional person it was possible to raise objections with.

'Sorry,' she said. 'Look, maybe I'm not really the right person for this particular type of problem. Tell you what, my supervisor is much more experienced in your kind of thing. I'll give you her card, and you can contact her'. No mention was made of a refund.

I phoned the supervisor a couple of days later, and she sounded less than delighted to have her supervisee's problem handed over without prior discussion. Possibly expecting trouble, she took, and retained, the offensive.

'So, do you have epilepsy?'

'Epilepsy? Shouldn't think so. I've never had fits or anything.'

She breathed hard down the phone.

'But your doctor hasn't ruled it out?'

'Well, no.'

'That response to flashing lights sounds like epilepsy.'

'But surely only if I also had fits?'

'Epilepsy is a contraindication for hypnotherapy'.

There was a pause in which I worked out what 'contraindication' meant and considered saying that perhaps she should tell her supervisee to explain that on her leaflet, but she seized her advantage.

'I can only treat you if you provide medical evidence of not being epileptic.' Touché.

I blinked.

'You mean, go and ask my GP to test me for something I don't have the symptoms of?'

I could picture the scene, and began to feel quite sick. My GP already thought I was a time-waster.

'Tell you what,' I said. 'Why don't we just leave it there?'

She agreed that it was probably for the best.

And that was the end of the hypnotherapy saga. Three failures is enough, and I never tried again, except occasionally with a recording on YouTube which encourages a bit of harmless relaxation beside a bubbling stream. It is tantalising, though. I'm still pretty sure that in the right hands, with the right script, it would have helped.

Mamma Mia

I AM A fully-paid-up psychotherapist these days, and I wonder if my urge to start that expensive and arduous training germinated from seeds sown by these three people who showed me the hard way that if therapies are to help, they have to speak the client's language, and not just the therapist's. They also left me with a sense that it would be a relief, perhaps even helpful in itself, to describe my experience to somebody willing and able to listen properly, though I didn't believe this strongly enough to actually look into talking therapies. But as it turned out, an unexpected and deeply unwelcome set of circumstances decreed that my next therapeutic foray was into the world of counselling.

I was still working in the civil service when it started. My phone rang one lunchtime. My colleagues and I never went out together, but we took out our sandwiches at the same time and chatted, or read our papers and novels. Tim and I were engaged in a cultural swap for which I had to plough through the meaty science fiction he favoured, flinching at the violent bits, while he tackled his first ever Jane Austen. Tim was forever doing things for the first time. He had moved out of his parents' home by now and got his own flat with a double bed, whereupon nature had taken its course with a woman he met in his new local, thereby changing the tone of the office banter, to the relief, I think, of all three of us.

My phone rang. I put down my Ursula Le Guin, and it was Mum, hoping it wasn't an inconvenient time. There was a bit of throat-clearing, then:

'Darling, you know I had a bit of jaundice, and they were going to do tests.'

'Yes?'

She spoke again, but I had to shush Tim, who was hooting at 'Catherine began to curl her hair and long for balls'.

'What did you say, Mum?'

'Some kind of autoimmune disease, in my liver. I thought I should let you know.'

I felt more bewildered than anything. Mum had always prided herself on her excellent health. 'Just a cold,' she would say each winter, shaking and shivering. 'I've never been one to catch flu'.

'Oh,' I said. 'Oh dear. Well, I hope you feel better soon. What happens next?'

That is how it started. I went home to see her; she was cheerful and matter of fact. She answered my questions about her prognosis (two to five years), and as the months went by, she let me know about her subsequent appointments at the hospital. There were recurring, hideous tests involving needles in her liver, the mildest description of which made me feel faint. Her blood and vital organs were monitored, monitored, monitored every month or week. As far as I could see, this macabre data gathering was entirely for its own sake, because they could offer no treatment. In her place, I would have refused the tests, perhaps underlining my point with a kick in the stomach. But she didn't. With the doctors and nurses and support staff, even with the researchers who gave her a placebo in a drug trial, she was polite, considerate, even grateful, to the end. Rodney would have been proud of her. I know I was.

The end was a liver transplant, the single arrow in their quiver of remedies, held back as long as possible because, as the doctor explained to Mum and she to me, the surgery was new, and unlikely to work. It didn't, or not for long. Three days of rosier skin were followed by two of sepsis and one on life support. Prometheus would have counted the operation an act of grace. By that time, I did too.

I had never imagined how close she and I really were, under all the non-communication. We never found out much about each other's inner worlds, but during the five years it took her to die (she was a true Rodney, following every instruction, trusting in the outcomes, even when fatal; she took the years allotted, not a day more) – during those five years, I recognised, and delighted in, and mourned in advance, the intense, mutual love and appreciation that lay beneath our silence.

In the fourth of Mum's five years, I left the civil service to start a two year residential course at a Bible College which specialised in training overseas missionaries. It seems now a surprising thing to have done, and possibly more connected with Mum's illness than I realised at the time. True, I was a mainstream believer in those days, to the mild surprise of my parents who had no interest at all in such matters, even negative. Mum and Dad hadn't been bothered when I started going to church, unprovoked, in my teens, though I did catch her staring at me one day as she mused:

'I was just wondering where on earth you get it from,

darling, this religious stuff – nobody else in the family has ever been like that.'

Mum's indifference only morphed into antipathy when I announced my intention of leaving the civil service, cashing in my pension (God, I regret that now) and renting out my flat to pay for the course.

'Bible College! What the hell is a Bible College? How can you spend two years studying one book?'

I could only reply at the time that it felt like the right thing to do. I was not finding the Civil Service particularly meaningful, especially since getting promoted and being moved to a data security section which was staffed by a tiny and dispirited group of oddballs, none of whom had much idea what data security was or how it was effected. We spent our days liaising with a team of expensive consultants who were doing the actual work, and most of my time went on activities like filling in my timesheet, arranging my pens on my desk and, if I was lucky, a bit of photocopying. I begged for some kind of training, but my line manager only came up with a week's Telecommunications course describing the types of wiring used in various networks, and the means by which they each transmitted 'packets' of code. After five days of uncomprehending boredom, I did not repeat my request.

So the months went gloomily by. The only positive things were that I could still walk to work and that doing nothing was easy on the eyesight, though possibly not on the mental health. Every now and then I would ask if there was any way at all that I could take on some aspect of the work covered by the consultants, but my boss would shake his head and advise:

'Best not to do anything. If you don't do anything, you can't get into trouble.'

I think now that he might have been clinically depressed. He never got in to work before 11, and I never saw him smile.

So I left the job, and left London for a life in a converted mansion in Hertfordshire. I have to say that if I had been deliberately seeking a place in which to endure my mother's final illness, it was a good choice. There were things to occupy your time, but it didn't matter much if you didn't feel up to them – lectures, workshops, a bit of socialising at so-called 'coffee parties', practical work around the college. Washing up. 'Veg prep'. None of it was particularly taxing on the eyesight or brain, but if there was any problem, there was always somebody ready to help. I'm not keen on institutional life, and it wouldn't have suited me at any other time, but it was a godsend then.

I've been lucky in my life to mostly encounter the best sort of Christianity, the loving-kindness type, and there were buckets of sympathy available for a twenty-something daughter in the last stages of losing her fifty-something mother. Perhaps for the first time, something that bothered me was striking a chord with those around me. The staff and students were endlessly patient in listening to whatever I wanted to say about Mum, but my tutor suggested that counselling would be a good thing too, and offered to recommend someone.

Unfortunately the counselling service she suggested was run by the sort of Christian outfit which I have always preferred to avoid: socially homogenous, self-satisfied, us-and-them-based. I feel like apologising for being so rude, but there is no point in pretending that I feel any kind of affinity with all or even most religious/spiritual organisations. More about all this later.

So I was introduced to Madeleine, I think her name was, who worked from a chilly pre-fab behind a church hall. The space was absolutely without character, but it was private and had a view of trees and did not contain the dreaded examination couch and desk. There was barely space for two armchairs and a small coffee table bearing a packet of Kleenex. Next to the tissues stood a wooden box with a peeling label saying 'Donations', which I regret to say I pretended not to see.

Madeleine, white-haired and smartly-buttoned with a patent leather handbag and matching shoes, seemed confident enough, and she could certainly do all the nodding and hmm-ing and putting the head on one side that became familiar to me in later therapists. I expect I do all that too, and I didn't have to learn the head tilting. I don't know how much training she'd had, if any, but I am sure that like the hypnotherapists and indeed the NHS, she meant well. I wonder now if she had a touch of undiagnosed dementia. There is nothing us-and-them about mental health problems.

'And do you have any brothers or sisters?' she asked every week, leaving me wondering what she thought I had been talking about when I explained, at her request, my family's composition and how Mum related to each of us. I lost myself in her questions. 'How is it…?' 'When did you…?' 'What are you…?' I cannot recall gaining a single insight, or feeling in any way comforted, or experiencing any relief in being able to talk about myself, only frustration that once again I had failed to make contact. And yet, as with the hypnotherapy, I retained some faith in the process itself that led me to try again, and again.

To be fair, I only saw Madeleine, if that was her name,

three or four times. She went on holiday, and while she was away, my mother died. I sent a note letting her know when I'd be back from the funeral so that we could arrange another appointment, and she responded with a sympathy card, a white and silver cross in moonlight, with an improbable background of lilies. It said:

'Let me know when you are ready to come again. You will need some time to get over your mother's death'.

Oh! And there was me thinking that people had counselling because they were unhappy. It is a shame that that card arrived at one of the rare times in my life where I could not raise a laugh. I wish I had it now.

Faith, Hope and Osteopathy

FAITH IS A not bad word for my continuing sense, in the teeth of Annie, Yin, Lucy and Madeleine, that the world of alternative treatments and talking therapies was the place for me, and that conventional medicine was best avoided. The events of the next few years affirmed both positions.

As well as Faith and Hope I had also acquired Desperation, that great incentive for trying new things. Mum's loss had literally crushed me, and every symptom that developed during my twenties was now magnified. A disc in my lower back kept slipping. My ankles kept turning over and spraining. My head appeared to have been rammed into my spine, causing one of my ribs to pop out. Even my wrists ached, and my big toes.

And so began the Osteopathy phase. There were plenty to choose from in London, and I cast my net wide, but as with doctors, the actual appointments didn't vary much. The practitioner would take a history, which was rather a lengthy business involving some bemusement about my eye condition ('You mean, they don't know what caused it?'). When the examination started, they would poke a cautions finger into my neck ('Good God, what on earth have you been doing?') and apply some form of massage, at some level between uncomfortable and excruciating. Occasionally they did that thing where they tie you up with your own arms and punch you in the ribs until something snaps. ('Now,' said lovely Irish Thomas as he took my trembling hands in his, 'This will be extremely painful, so I want you to relax completely'.)

After half an hour or so, they would step back, and I would find that I could move freely. I would leap off the couch, babble my thanks, write a cheque and set off home, swinging my arms or rotating my neck or whatever I had been unable to do previously. And by the end of the day I would be in agony again, and either make a follow-up appointment or go back to the directory.

It was a grim business, the repeated free-falling slide from hope to agony. What on earth was going wrong? No knives or drugs were involved, so it couldn't be the same thing that went wrong with conventional medicine, and these new folk made no assaults on my subconscious mind as the hypnotherapists had done. These practitioners were all qualified, with good reputations and full waiting rooms, but what they offered was never right for me. A few of them were actually recommended by people I trusted. 'Oh, that Thomas, you won't believe what he did for my knee; I hadn't walked for a year, but after one treatment I danced the cancan all night' kind of thing. I started to feel nervous, almost guilty, in the presence of anyone who swore by these treatments. What would her name be, somebody universally enthusiastic about alternatives? Gwyneth, perhaps.

Given my physical state, it was fortunate that the stint at Bible College did not result in the overseas pioneering work

I had vaguely imagined signing up for. Something about spending two years entirely with evangelical Christians, kind though they were, had put me right off identifying as an officially spiritual person; I was not even as keen as I had been on God. Indeed, I essayed a whole first draft of this book without mentioning my time at the college, but my draft readers complained that they couldn't follow the story without it.

Anyway, instead of hacking my way short-sightedly through the jungle, I was back in my South London flat, working in database development for a charity, and getting paid reasonably well. A good part of my salary went on physical treatments, and I added a talking therapist or two to my staff list. I found Robin through another low-cost pastoral organisation, and was relieved to find that he charged a fixed rate, so I didn't have to avoid the eye of the donations box. Even better, Robin helped, a bit. He was the one who made me realise I'd been angry with my parents about the eye operations, which was hard to accept because (I would say now) accepting that your mother has let you down is usually hard, especially at that stage of bereavement where you can see no wrong in the departed, who you feel deserves to be defended even unto your own death.

I saw Robin weekly for a few months, and stopped not so much because I was ready, as because we had an argument about a wardrobe. This probably sounds very silly, but a lot of what happens in therapy sounds silly until you understand what is behind it. Robin had a wardrobe in his consulting room, a vast object about nine feet high and four feet wide, its little fat legs crouched as though in readiness to scuttle away. Its grainy side surface was the first thing to greet me when I entered the room, so that I almost had to walk into it – through it – in order to reach Robin, the back of whose chair rested against the slippery face of its doors. Was Robin protecting the wardrobe, or vice versa?

This item of furniture became something of an obsession for me, of more interest than my own life or anything that Robin might say about it. I speculated about it endlessly, both during and between appointments, even in my sleep. It was far too big for the size of the room, seeming at least as wide as the doorway. How did it get in there in the first place? Was the building perhaps constructed around it; had it been there since the beginning of time?

Robin sat with his back to the wardrobe, and I sat facing the two of them, and wondered about them both. Was Robin homeless, and living in his consulting room? Did he climb into the wardrobe after I went home, and remain until the following week? I realise now that it took me back to the hauntings, imagined or otherwise, of my earliest years, heavy oak furniture being a feature of my family home, and these infantile imaginings were a natural result.

I didn't understand that then, but I knew the wardrobe had some significance and kept trying to bring the conversation round to it and its contents, while Robin became increasingly irritated, finally snapping: 'This is my room, and I have what I want in it'. I felt hurt at this dismissal, and also suspected that he wasn't supposed to say things like that, so I gave him notice. He didn't believe I meant it, and was bewildered when I shook his hand and wished him well two weeks later. In a way it was a shame, because he was helping me, and I wish now that I had hung on in there and tried to explain, or that he had realised it meant something and explored it a bit.

So much for the psyche. Back in the soma, I was giving

chiropractic a try (too violent), then reflexology (gave me leg cramps), then Bowen Technique (ouch). Different modalities; same temporary relief followed by worse pain. Gwyneth despaired, and suggested I just go to a class if I was that hard to please, so I tried Pilates with several different teachers. How could Pilates have the same effect as the treatments? Well, it did. The first teacher refused to have me in her class because when she 'checked in' at the beginning of each evening by asking us all whether we'd had any physical problems after the previous week, I kept on telling her. After that, I tried a new teacher and a policy of keeping quiet, but with no better results. Gwyneth started to suspect I was taking the piss, and Rodney couldn't see why I wouldn't stop wasting my money and go to see Louise, the NHS physiotherapist who was so good when he broke his leg.

I am racing through the years now; these episodes did not follow each other as closely as it sounds. That really would be masochism... No; I would try something out, get scared and leave it for a few months, until some crisis, the slipped disc usually, sent me thumbing the directories.

But things started to look up psyche-wise. A friend introduced me to a psychotherapist called Jennifer, who charged exactly twice as much as Robin and was worth it. She said once, when I was cringing after somebody shouted at me for failing to see a bicycle zooming along the pavement, 'You get upset when people treat you as if you're stupid because *you* fear you are stupid.' Obvious once you know, but a revelation at the time. Jennifer's tolerance of intrusive remarks was also proportional to her fees. I remember for some reason describing the appearance of a particularly badly-dressed colleague – corduroy pinafore dress, tan-coloured tights and Scholl sandals – and realising that actually it was Jennifer who was sporting that outfit, even as we spoke. She realised at the same moment, and gave me the most beatific, comforting smile.

So things were improving with the talking therapy, and then, after about ten years of trying, came a breakthrough on the physical front. I feel strange admitting this, almost as though my job, perhaps my life purpose, is to be The One Whom No Treatment Helps. ('A one' in fact. There are plenty like me. Yes, there are, Rodney and Gwyneth). The tide turned, first gently, then in a rush. First I met Elaine. Then I met Miranda. Then I met Drew. And then, the grand finale, I met Guillermo. But in the centre of this flowering meadow of healing, there festered a deadly swamp. The Lumbarjack episode.

I'm A Lumbarjack And I'm OK (Monty Python, 1969)

ELAINE WAS AN osteopath working 'in the cranial field'. This was a new term to me, and one I came to revere, along with 'cranial-sacral'. She turned out to be the last of my series of London–based practitioners, not because I had given the whole thing up as hopeless and gone away to shoot myself, but because I needed to look no further. Elaine worked from a local clinic which offered a variety of therapies, and had ergo been the scene of several painful incidents over the years. The worse of these involved an over-enthusiastic neck massage followed by a total blackout in the waiting room. The woman on reception was close to calling an ambulance, but first consulted the masseuse, who went pale and hazarded that the cause of my indisposition was an inadequate breakfast. Huh! I lacked the energy to contest the breakfast theory, and anyway, what facts did I have to support my furious conviction that a banana and milky coffee were sufficient for a morning's bus-ride followed by a lie-down on a couch? Anyway, did I really want to accuse this bewildered woman of injuring me, based on unscientific gut instinct?

And so it was that the clinic, housed above a Victorian shop on a main road, already reverberated with anxious vibes of my own, and my heart as I climbed the stairs to Elaine's room was head-heavy. Turning the handle of the door, I was unsurprised to find a tiny space, a treatment couch almost touching the edge of a wooden desk, and beside it that familiar patient's chair at exactly the worst angle for my null point. I noticed these things, but I noticed something else too. A venetian-blinded window conveying cheery, dappled daylight, and beside it a young oval face, dark-haired, dark-eyed, that beamed out professional interest softened with humorous compassion.

'Have a seat,' said Elaine, 'while I sort out a fresh index card.'

And without even thinking, let alone asking or explaining, I twirled around the patient's chair to face her.

I cannot describe the relief of finally explaining my symptoms to somebody to whom they made sense. 'Yes,' she said, turning her own neck this way and that, 'your head tilt would throw out *this* and put pressure on *that*…' I can't remember the exact words. She knew about nystagmus, even that it was not the same thing as astigmatism, which I also had. In this, she did better than most of the other osteopaths, and won hands down over a certain nurse at Moorfields who took down my medical history when I went in with a minor injury, and for whom I had to define 'nystagmus' as well as spell it.

I trusted Elaine about three minutes into our conversation, and when it was time for the treatment, the couch yielded to my already relaxing spine. 'I'll just work gently for now,' she said, and laid a careful hand for minutes at a time on my head, then under my hip, then over my foot. And throughout my body, things moved, strengthened, released, hurt briefly, then recovered. I told her what was going on, and she smiled with white, even, natural teeth, and said that most patients didn't feel so much with this type of work, just knew they felt better afterwards.

'Your system is very sensitive,' she said. 'It is sensitive anyway, but also the body can only stand so much misalignment before something gives. You are at the end of your compensation'.

I was at the end of my compensation! I would never have thought of putting it like that, but the moment she said it, it became deeply true.

After that first treatment there was no backlash; I was calm, exhausted in fact, and slept for hours and hours, waking only to gulp water and sleep again. I am not saying that she cured me completely. I was still more easily unbalanced than most of my peer group, still subject to muscular problems. But over the next few months my periods of comfort and cheer became longer than they had ever been, even before Mum's death. When something slipped or twisted, I went back for a session, usually just one, and felt better. Her approach was to work cautiously, doing the minimum possible, and quite often saying, when I was enjoying something and wanting more, 'I'm going to leave this for now, or you'll get a reaction later.' In time my whole system, accustomed to associate physical interventions with fear and shock, opened up and ran more smoothly. Oh, the relief, the gratitude.

Elaine turned out to live in the same road as me, and we got to know each other better through being neighbours. Both cat-lovers, we took on each other's cat feeding during holidays, and occasionally drank a cup of coffee together. I referred to Elaine any of my family and friends who found themselves in physical distress, including my partner, and when she attended our wedding reception years later, we found that she had treated most of the people at her table, including the priest who led the service.

It feels tragic now, that this period of unexpected wellbeing was the background to the lumbarjack episode. In my memory it was Steve, my now husband, then partner, who instigated it, though the suggestion still upsets him. Of course, being an adult of relatively sound mind, I was the one who signed the form.

Steve may have been a catalyst, but so was my lifelong tendency to fall over for no apparent reason, which recurred during this time with some unpleasant consequences. Twice I was walking around the house when my left foot seemed to freeze so that I toppled awkwardly, once twisting my wrist and once (Elaine said at the next appointment) spraining a rib. The third and worst instance happened at the railway station. I was moving to get on an approaching train, when I fell forward on the platform, almost pushing another commuter on to the track. It was scary stuff. I saw Elaine after each incident, and though she helped the injuries to heal, her treatments did not seem to address the cause of the random unsteadiness.

Steve was anxious.

'Claire, this is madness; you could be killed; you have to see a doctor.'

'Not seeing a doctor. They only make things worse.'

'For God's sake, just make an appointment, or I'll make it, do you want me to go with you?'

Despite all I had told him, and looking back perhaps I had not told him enough, Rodney remained convinced that my doctor phobia was down to illogical fear, not bitter experience. Did I say Rodney? Steve, I meant to say, though at that time he was a true Rodney in all but name. When *Steve* found it too painful to walk, he was diagnosed with Morton's Neuroma and fixed with a steroid injection. When *Steve* got a nasty growth on his head, the potion provided by the GP removed it without causing the side effects whose details I read out, wide-eyed, begging him to stick the stuff in the bin.

Interestingly, Steve was the son of the most ardent non-Rodney I have ever met. Apart from minimum contact when producing her four children, my mother-in-law had had no truck with the medical profession since she was hospitalised as a child with a mysterious skin disease that was never diagnosed. An isolation hospital, it was, and they kept her there for months, watching her and doing the odd test. Eventually she recovered on her own and was allowed home, and that was it, for her, as far as medicine went. She included dentistry in her embargo, pulling out her own teeth when they hurt and, when they were all gone, squeezing into her late husband's dentures.

I rather admired this attitude; it was something we had in common; but Steve and his brothers were not impressed.

'If you're ill, you go to the doctor,' they would say, and Steve said it loudest of all, shaking his head at my repeated injuries.

I gave in eventually, mostly because it felt unkind to keep refusing. I signed on at a local practice where the GP spent eight minutes hitting my knees with hammers and telling me to stand on one leg or touch my nose with my finger, then referred me for what was charmingly called 'a battery of tests'. They certainly battered me. He must have been concerned about me, because the appointments were arranged within the month. Blood tests, which showed nothing, and then a lumbar puncture. I arranged an appointment with Elaine the day before this procedure, hoping this would set me up to be relaxed and in good fettle for what I expected would be an ordeal. When I told her this, she said 'Mmfff,' and was rather quiet for the rest of the session, but asked me before I left to let her know how it went.

My heart and my stomach are already churning at the prospect of writing this, so I'll be brief.

At the hospital, they gave me a bed on the top floor overlooking a park, and this made me feel a bit safer, quashing my rising desire to refuse to sign the form and go home. But I did sign the form.

A young doctor turned up at the appointed hour and said that he had to get the registrar to come and watch him do the procedure, so we waited still longer. It was August, and very likely he was on his first rotation, and had not done this before.

Whatever this man did, with the other man watching him, took quite a long time. I can't remember the detail. The young doctor told me to keep my head down afterwards 'or you might get a headache', so I rested on that bed by the window until dusk, when he let me go home in a taxi, reiterating the advice about lying down flat. I went straight to bed and stayed there until the following morning. I had the day off work, and didn't feel like getting up, so I lay in bed until lunchtime, but I didn't want any lunch.

Steve was due back from work at five o'clock, but at half past two I rang up asking him to come home at once. I was feeling so ill that I didn't want to be alone in the house in case I started to die. I had never felt so ill as this, nothing like it. Rigid, throbbing pain filled my head and seeped right down my neck. My nystagmus was going so fast that the room reeled and swam. Light exploded round the edge of the blackout curtain although the day was cloudy. My ears were screeching with tinnitus, my throat palpating with nausea. I remembered about keeping my head down, and was too dizzy to stand anyway, so I crawled to the bathroom with my head hanging low.

Steve, when he arrived home, was horrified; I had seemed fine, just a bit sleepy, when he'd gone out. Pretty much immobilised by pain, I asked him to ring the hospital and find out if this was normal. He couldn't get through at first, so he googled. 'Severe lumbar puncture syndrome', he found, with an exact list of my symptoms. The hospital eventually answered their phone and somebody, for all I know a receptionist or a cleaner, told Steve that yes, a headache was to be expected after that procedure, sometimes a bad one, and if he was really worried, the registrar who oversaw the procedure would ring back in the morning. Just keep lying down, and the headache would be gone in a couple of days.

A couple of days!

Steve rang Elaine next, and she said not to worry, these kind of symptoms often affected women who'd had epidurals, and she should be able to help. She came round in the morning, and my faith that she would make this better led me to raise my head a few inches, whereupon yellow vomit seeped thinly between my lips. I hardly cared. While Steve changed the pillow slips, she treated my back. Maybe she made a bit of difference. Or maybe it was just comforting to see her and to know that she was on my side.

The grim truth was that not even Elaine could unwind the effects of such a physical assault in a single session. She could, however, see how much pain I was in, and wondered aloud whether they had taken too much fluid from my spine, or whether fluid was leaking.

I am not a research scientist, but in my mind this experience is evidence for Elaine's treatments having a clinical value, not just a psychological one. I was all set up for a placebo effect, expecting and believing, indeed desperate, for a significant improvement, and it didn't happen.

As Elaine was saying goodbye the phone rang downstairs, and we heard Steve, obviously speaking to the registrar.

'Can you go down and ask about the fluid,' I managed to say.

Elaine buttoned her jacket and sighed.

'I'm not sure they would be willing to talk to me.'

Speaking from the hospital, the medical expert assured Steve that I probably had a virus unrelated to the lumbar puncture, that there was nothing he or his team could do, and that if I still felt poorly next week I should visit the GP. They had seriously ill patients to treat, and did not have time to discuss this further.

Up in my bedroom, Elaine accepted ten pounds for the treatment, to be paid when I felt better, and said she would do some research and be back the next day, which was a Sunday.

She left me with the pain. I forced down some ibuprofen, then paracetamol, but they made no difference. In the afternoon the emergency GP came to see me, reluctantly accepting Steve's insistence that I could not get to the surgery, being unable to stand. He gave me a huge injection of co-codamol which also made no difference. How could it have made no difference? I think Elaine said that the opioid receptors in the brain could only work properly with the spinal fluid at its correct level. Something like that. My concentration was not at its best.

I did get better eventually. I woke up about six days after that trip to the hospital recalling that once upon a time I used to brush my teeth in the mornings, and I found my toothbrush and used it, crouching in the bath. Some days later I was able to listen to a radio drama without the tinnitus drowning it out, then to sit up on the pillows for an hour or so. Gradually the 'headache' became a headache, then not even that. I began to visit Elaine in the clinic again, and went back to work.

That was the lumbarjack incident. The fire of my hatred of medical interventions, tamped for years, roared and spat anew. If *I* had made another human being that ill, I would want to know why, and how to avoid doing it to somebody else. Not so those experts at the hospital. They'd done their job and filled in their forms and were on to the next thing. The Lumbarjacks were OK.

Routine tests; testing routines.

I AM A practising psychotherapist these days, not a furious child. Not a demented harpy. Not a vengeful psychopath. Well, I am all of these things too, of course, and more, and sometimes one of them gets control of my mouth, or the keyboard. The reader may have observed my frequent nods throughout this work to the good intentions of those who tormented me, and this represents a part of me that hopes to be taken seriously by professionals as a reasonably rational, reasonably reasonable human being, who, when she suggests that not all medical tests and treatments are worth the candle, just might be saying something worth taking notice of.

Meanwhile, a little part of me is still screeching, red-faced and square-mouthed, at the casual, white-coated cruelty of that mean, nasty, *stupid* trick that made my life for a time not worth living, and might have killed me. The red-faced one is incapable of rational discussion, so it lies with a more grown up, though still livid, version of myself to fume that that completely useless so-called 'test' destabilised my brain and musculoskeletal system just at the point where I had found the first person ever to genuinely help me, and moreover that that person, who had studied for five years and continued to attend courses and to consult literature on exactly the sort of problem that I was experiencing, and who was not free at the point of delivery but was paid gladly by myself and others she helped, this professional in every sense, this godsend with a smile, was regarded by a crew of needle-happy medics as so inferior as to be not even worth speaking to on the phone.

When I hear, and I do hear, often, about other 'tests' with catastrophic 'side effects', being carried out in their thousands every year, I screech louder. I particularly loathe the invasive procedures, like mine, that are carried out 'in case' they show up anything useful. I wish I'd thought to ask what they hoped to discover from my lumbar puncture; how could they have answered?

'Oh, nothing special. Don't mind us. Just browsing'.

I loathe the way that certain procedures are described as 'routine' as though this means that the patient has nothing to worry about. Routine for the doctors and nurses and technicians, is what you mean. Things *you* do all day every day. Nothing complicated, that might force you to think about the patient as an individual, and wonder how they might be affected if, to pull an example out of the air, they are *already* showing signs of neurological imbalances *before* you upset the pressure in their brain by syphoning off their spinal fluid. Routine for you! Not so routine for the poor sod who doesn't know when they'll next be lifting their head.

Because it isn't just me, you know. Google Severe Lumbar Puncture Syndrome and you'll find loads of anecdotal evidence that it isn't that uncommon. Or just ask around. Only last week a friend told me of a colleague who, weeks after receiving a lumbar puncture, is still on sick leave, flat on her back with an agonising headache. She's been told that her wound did not heal up 'as it does in 99% of cases', but is still leaking spinal fluid. There will be an operation to repair it; she is on the waiting list; but she has been warned that this may not cure the headache.

Rodney is gulping a bit. 'Still, you were falling over and all that, and this procedure got them some useful information which helped you get better, right?'

No, Rodney, it didn't. They sent me a letter saying that the results were inconclusive and that they would need to do it again.

'You're joking, right?'

I'm not joking, Rodney. Still, ha ha, it was just a routine test, so why would I object to having it done again?

Rodney frowns; he doesn't like sarcasm.

'If it was really as bad as you say, maybe you should have complained.'

Well, I did. I complained to the hospital and to a patient liaison service who offered to get the quality of the information leaflet improved, but had no truck with my suggested wording: 'Severe lumbar puncture syndrome is commoner than most doctors think, and the procedure may easily yield no useful results, so think twice before agreeing'. The liaison service made a milder suggestion, and I gave up. Couldn't stand thinking about it any more.

My effort at complaining had been half-hearted, but I was nervous about having complained at all, fearing that the next time I went to see my GP, which I hoped would not be for many decades, the doctor would hold it against me. Fortunately nothing like that happened, because they kept no record of my having complained at all, or of my having had a bad experience with the lumbar puncture. My notes said that I'd had a codeine injection the day after the procedure, and as they'd heard nothing else, they assumed I was fine. It was just a routine test, after all.

I loathe everything about routine tests. I loathe all the mistakes; all the positives which come out negative, and all the 'false positives' which helter-skelter the patient from test to test until good news is confirmed. 'Congratulations on being fine after all. Pop back in November, and we'll do it all again'.

I loathe the whole production line of fear; those women in terror of their next smear or mammogram, those old men waiting to hear if they have bowel cancer, peering into the toilet bowl, in search of blood.

I loathe the barefaced Conventional Medical cheek that dismisses the successes of the likes of Elaine as 'placebo effect' whilst disregarding the reverse-placebo effects in which they themselves covertly specialise. Do you never wonder, Doctors, about the drip-drip-drip effect of your questions? 'Have you got bowel cancer yet?' 'Have you got heart disease yet?' 'Have you got cervical cancer yet, or prostate?' If what you say about placebo is true, and people get better because they expect to, surely all this focus on alarming symptoms must be making people more likely to feel, or fall, ill? If you are right when you say that patients feel better after alternative treatments because the practitioner listens to them and seems to care, why is not listening and not seeming to care so very, very normative in conventional medicine?

I'm going too far now, and Rodney is shaking his head. He's just pleased that his mum's breast cancer was diagnosed early and that she's well again.

I'm glad too, Rodney, but we don't know what price she paid in the process. We also don't know how many other women now have cancer because of the same test that diagnosed your mum; mammograms can *cause* cancer, did you know that? No, I've lost him; he doesn't want to hear this stuff. I'm banging my head against a brick wall, most of the time. No wonder I feel dizzy.

I feel dizzy now. I have to remind myself that whilst acknowledging and accepting the presence of one's inner voices is important, so is finding ways to calm down. One thing Elaine did for my system was to help it enjoy a sense of balance. Her treatments were not the only example of that, and now is the time to say more about what helped in this way. And, inevitably, what did not.

False starts seem to be the story of my life, and just as I made one with therapy, so I did with yoga. The year after the lumbarjack incident, Steve and I, both feeling for different reasons a need to stretch and relax, signed up for a weekly class.

Iyenga for Beginners, as it was called, was taught by a woman called Jill, assisted by her partner, Bruno. The class took place in a church hall with a very dirty floor. The available space was long and thin, and the class popular, so we students laid out our mats close together in two long rows. Jill insisted on perfect alignment of mat as well as body, so the first minutes of each class were spent tugging at corners. Our blankets and straps, when not in use, had to be folded and placed on the outer edges of our mats. It was a bit like being in the army.

Jill tended to give a lightning demo of each posture before prowling the hall to pounce on mistakes, and she was mostly positioned way beyond the scope of my detail-vision.

My ability to grasp what was required at first relied on the expertise of the student on my left, until I explained about my eyesight and balance issues, whereupon Jill became alarmingly positive.

'Don't you worry about that. Bruno will help you!'

So when the command came to stand on one leg, or to form some triangular shape beyond my competence, Bruno would come marching through the ranks. His idea of helping was to get a good grip on various parts of my anatomy and yank them into the arrangement prescribed by Jill. Because he was a big strong chap and I didn't like to make a fuss, he usually succeeded. Whether it was yoga in any normal sense, was another question. I certainly came out of that class with some unfamiliar muscular sensations, but whilst appreciating, as usual, the intention behind the rugby tackle, I did not find it particularly relaxing.

Steve was rather jealous of Bruno's attentions, not for romantic reasons but because he could have done with some help himself. He was one of three men in that class; less supple than the women, they tended to gather together for support, enabling Jill to admonish them in one breath.

'Come on, you old stiffies, straighten those legs'.

Steve posed no objection when I suggested a change of class. Jill had her place on the prestigious Iyenga Register, but a certain handwritten advert, flapping in a newsagent's window, had its own appeal. When we turned up for the new class in a school hall, only the dirty floor struck a chord. A smaller number of mats were set out in a semi-circle in front of a wavy-haired figure in red trousers, whose eyes were closed, deep in meditation. This was Miranda, and as with Elaine, meeting her felt like coming home.

Doing Miranda's sort of yoga, my body found the

releasing and stretching that I now realised it craved. There was lots of lying down flat – good - and making gentle rocking movements – good - and lying with your legs up the wall to take the pressure off your spine – excellent. As soon as I mentioned neck problems, I was let off a whole raft of challenges, instead being authorised by Miranda to rest in well-aligned peace, whilst all around me Steve and the others struggled to stand on their heads or their hands. There was a lot of laughter in that class; Jill would have been astonished. That first evening, Miranda got us to lie on our backs with our feet right over our heads, before announcing in sepulchral tones: 'Beware: this is known as The Wind Release Position' and collapsing into giggles. Jill would have been scandalised.

And there was a long, long relaxation at the end, in which Miranda's voice rocked us to the depths of bliss.

I soon discovered that Miranda offered alternative treatments too: reiki and Indian head massage, though she confided that she was giving up the latter because it was too much like hard work. I went for a session of reiki, and even if no other benefit had resulted, it would have been enough to lie quietly in her high-windowed house, gorgeous with silk rugs and paintings and flowers, and to feel Miranda's warm hands close to, not even touching, my body. Her presence recalled Elaine's expansive gentleness, though Miranda did not talk in terms of anatomy or physiology. Instead she had an eclectic and fascinating set of beliefs that could be loosely classed as 'spiritual'.

I had never met anyone like Miranda. As I had more treatments, and did more yoga, and found the courage to ask her to lunch, and was asked back with Steve to meet her family, and found a beloved, hilarious friend who never failed to raise my spirits, I continued intrigued at the things she said, casually, in the midst of chat about her cat or the price of soya. She believed that time was speeding up, and would soon reach a point where it no longer existed, so we would be doing everything at the same moment. She was looking forward to the day when the most enlightened human beings would be moved to a new version of our planet. ('But how will that be for the rest of us?' 'Oh, the others won't notice. Replicas of the missing people will be left behind.'). I valued her opinions, however outlandish, because she was usually right, in essence, on important matters. She was sending healing energy into the oceans long before there was serious concern about pollution, and she could explain her friends' behaviour in terms of their past lives, with great astuteness. And the practices she taught, I have to say, worked, in much the way that prayer can work, whatever you think about God. 'Drawing down the violet flame' for instance – that was powerful.

Steve, on the whole less open to this kind of thing, liked her as much as I did, and to keep the conversation going without compromising his own integrity, he developed a habit of saying 'Sorry, Miranda; I can't follow you there,' which made her laugh. Her husband, a successful businessman with a wonderful bass voice, would growl at her to shut up ('they'll think you're mad, darling!'), and that made her laugh even more, leaning back and pouring wine and beaming at the company.

Just being with Miranda was healing, but I believed in the reiki too. I was sure by now that healing could happen with gentle laying on of hands, and that Miranda, for all her unexpected ideas, was a master of her craft. No side effects, either.

From Flake to Ferrari

I'M NOT SOUNDING very robust, am I, falling at the consecutive fences of Level 1 Pilates and Beginners Yoga, only to collapse unconscious from a relaxing massage. Some people will be suspecting that I am a bit of a snowflake. Although this modern term of abuse mainly applies to folk who express themselves offended – devastated, even - by any opinion that they disagree with, the word also applies to anyone who is 'sensitive' in any area of life, and I cannot deny that I come into this category.

Some snowflakes have had a go at reclaiming the concept, suggesting that it indicates political awareness or solidarity with the oppressed, but nobody buys that. Snowflakes may look pretty but they are, frankly, too easily crushed to be useful. Pour cold water on the opinions, and they dissolve. Press them and they turn to mush. Flakes are 'sensitive' and require 'sensitivity' from others, but somehow they are fated not to receive it. They annoy other people, that is the brutal truth. The content of their objections, which may be perfectly valid, is lost; their reasonable requests for reasonable adjustments are scorned.

So it is with some trepidation that I describe my brain and body as 'sensitive', but I can think of no better word.

'Highly-strung'? 'Finely-tuned'? 'Delicate'? Oh, no! The best I can think of is 'misaligned', which sounds more neutral and less likely to demand unreasonably special treatment. But 'misaligned' does not convey how quickly I slip into physical distress in response to certain experiences: drugs, uncomfortable chairs, transport, people sitting on my right and so on. I am also suggestible, ridiculously so; I have been known to retch just *listening to a description* of a speeding coach on winding roads. Sensitivity gone mad.

I am not proud of any of this, but I don't want to be ashamed of it either. Being sensitive is no fun, and neither is having to choose between experiencing, and being, a pain. Ooh, something is not exactly right for me, poor me; everybody must get up and move around, until I am perfectly comfortable.

Personally, I'd like to take all the value judgement out of the word ; not just the negatives, but 'sensitive' as in 'special', and use it as a straightforward descriptor. Whenever my disc slips while I'm on holiday, which it usually does because hotel mattresses are too soft (princess-and-the-pea, but in reverse), I'd like to be able to say unselfconsciously to the local osteopath: 'My system is very sensitive. Please take account of that.' Instead, I have to get them on the phone and ask leading questions until they give themselves away, or not. 'Ooh, you'd be surprised how much pressure the body can tolerate,' said one cheerful soul who did not make it past an initial enquiry.

There was just one person who successfully challenged my sensitivity. This was not a doctor or an alternative therapist, but, of all people, an Argentinian Tango maestro and voice coach.

I'd always longed to sing well, but I was one of millions

who were told at the age of four that I was out of tune, and then kept my mouth shut in perpetuity. Tragic! But some time in my forties, bolstered by the good energy from Elaine and Miranda and others, I decided to try again. I looked for a local singing teacher on the website of something called the Natural Voice Network. The site was full of encouraging phrases like 'If you can speak, you can sing', and 'Singing is our birthright'. So I arranged a series of lessons with Guillermo, in an ex-council flat near the Elephant and Castle where I used to work with Tim and Phil, what seemed like centuries ago.

Oh Guillermo! I had never imagined I would follow anyone so quickly, so far from my comfort zone. Experience had taught me to preserve my fragile flakiness from the stomping boots of medical and alternative well-wishers, but you showed me that the most delicately crystalline structure has an inner heft of its own.

The day you took me to the park and made me sing, on a rising note, spread-eagled on the grass amidst staring passers-by and bemused alcoholics, a resounding 'LA-GAR, LA-GAR, LA-GAR'!

The way you stood me facing the window of your room and said 'Look at the horizon. No, look with both eyes. I know, but your inner body has two eyes; look with them. That's better!' And my neck and head steadied, and I felt huge and wonderful, and when I sang my voice was rich and full!

The day I just couldn't seem to breath properly, and my song was laboured and low, and you inquired rather brusquely, 'What the fuck was that?'. And my eyes filled with tears, and you said, 'No, don't get all sensitive, breathe,' and I thought 'Oh – OK then', and, astoundingly, I stepped away from the hurt feelings into a deep, beautiful breath which emerged as a steady hum. 'Respiration is inspiration', you reminded me. And it was.

The way you said, 'Find your inner flow, and sing from there. Not like that. Why should I listen?' You turned your back and said 'I will look round when you engage me'. And after much muttering, I found my inner flow and sang strongly, and you whirled around, and your smiling eyes met mine!

The way you gave me so much pure gold that I set aside my snowflake-self who might have been wounded, and my professional self who might have condemned, when you rearranged my lesson at short notice, then rearranged again. The day that you were hungry when I arrived, and you cooked, and ate, a fried egg, licking your fingers and twanging your guitar, and I carried on regardless.

And thus you challenged my snowflake sensitivity, not by denying or dismissing it but by speaking to some inner robustness that had been there, I soon realised, all along. All the time there was a well-balanced, level-headed woman with a powerful voice just waiting to get out, and it was you, Guillermo, who made the introduction, in our very first lesson, where you heard me sing a few bars and said, 'Hmmm. You drive yourself like a clapped-out Ford, when you are really a brand new Ferrari.

74

Song For Ali

It is so strange that I was planning to write more about singing today anyway, about singing and how it helps, about how it is taught and experienced and lived, and about the friends I found through singing. I was going to muse about what a metaphor the voice can be for so many areas of life, speaking or singing, solo or in harmony.

Even Rodney is quite interested; he has been talking about what he calls 'the so-called benefits' of community choirs, which are so widely recommended just now. In the ten years since I discovered it, singing has come into fashion. Rodney isn't sure what to make of all this. He approves of the Military Wives Choir because he knows the women have a hard time and it seems to cheer them up, though he won't be drawn on how good he really thinks they sound. I suspect that he isn't sure how many other people need, or deserve, choral cheer. His boys go to band practice, but that's different. He doesn't expect them to be marching around tootling a trumpet in their mature years.

I was planning to say, today, that not every vocal coach is like Guillermo. I was going to say that there are many ways to lead a choir. Guillermo may actually be a one-off, with his ability to tune up a circle of choral novices to different pitches, two chanting, three humming, one yodelling, re-creating and adjusting and perfecting a toe-tingling joyride. Then there was his facility for bringing the sopranos (a notoriously chatty group) into attentive silence while the tenors were learning their parts… happy days.

Anyway. People are different. Today I was going to talk about Ali, eventually. I was going to talk about lots of other things first, but I don't want to now. It is just throat clearing.

We met Ali quite recently, after moving from London up to Cumbria three years ago. Perhaps the reader is engaged enough in my story to draw a breath at the thought of my leaving, all at once, the posse of therapists who made me feel better. But Steve and I both longed for fresh air and to be amongst beautiful countryside, and if we didn't do it now, in my fifties and his sixties, we might have felt too old. We didn't know anybody up here, and friends said we were 'brave', meaning 'stupid'. A pair of ageing Wordsworths, wandering like a couple of clouds.

So there we were, newly arrived in small town Cumbria, hundreds of miles not just from our friends and families and all those familiar therapists, but also from Guillermo, and from the leader who followed Guillermo in our home choir (Katy: gentle and laughing and on the side of the angels), and from raven-haired soprano Carollyn, and from the infinite musical choice that London offers. We joined our new town's Community Choir at first, which was nice, well led and inclusive, and a useful fount of local gossip. But I found it too big for comfort, and such hard work, peering at sheet music and sitting on uncomfortable chairs and always being at the wrong angle from the conductor, however much the kindly organisers allowed for 'reasonable adjustments'. We thirsted for the Natural Voice approach; small groups, standing or sitting as you liked, always able to move to the place you needed to be, physically and musically. No sheet music to hold close to your eyes, just the leader singing your part to you again and again until you got it.

So we found a Natural Voice practitioner leading a group some fifteen miles away, and began the process of enticing her closer. We kept turning up, or emailing or phoning, offering to sort out room bookings and do the publicity and manage the email list, and eventually she gave in and agreed to lead a group in our town hall on Wednesday afternoons. I printed out posters and learnt to laminate, Steve hung them on railings around the town.

And people came forward: mostly women, mostly middle aged, a sprinkling of younger people and even a few men. Marilyn and Anne and Kath and Daniel... I knew their names well from the list, though I struggled to put names to faces for an embarrassingly long time. I became sure first of Kath, a energetic lady with white hair and a young face, who would catch my eye and laugh about the way we both followed the movement of the tune with our hands. Disastrous when we were singing different parts, and watching each other's hands across the circle.

Anyway, the teacher we enticed was Ali. I need to talk about Ali. I can't talk about anything else today. I'm bored by my own ramblings. Never introduce! If you have something to say, say it.

What can I say about Ali? She was of medium height, with shiny dark hair in a bob and a big, dimpling smile. She could have been any age at all, but today I found out that she was 45 when we first met. She always wore leather boots or sandals, depending on the time of year, and harem pants with a loose shirt. She had a huge, resonant voice, very low for a woman; she could teach the bass parts in their own register. When she reached the sopranos, my part of choice, she would literally roll up her sleeves before singing the tune perfectly but lightly, then mopping her brow and urging us to take over.

Ali held the room. She was a gentle light dancing from place to place around the circle, and wherever she rested and beamed, the singers raised up their heads and opened their throats.

I was planning to tell Rodney, expounding on the benefits of song, that belonging to a choir offers the kind of discipline that is a relief to those who largely plan their own time. You pay the closest attention to the leader and the other singers, you listen, you do exactly what you're told, and the result, when practised and perfected, gives you complete happiness, and you see that joy reflected all round the circle, with Ali in the middle slowly revolving to face each of us, her hands held up, her mouth a little open, drinking in the harmony. Whether sharing the groundwork or reaping the harvest, your attention is absolutely absorbed; you think of nothing else. 'The complete, drug-free, sustainable antidote to depression and anxiety', I told Rodney once. He looked embarrassed. What tosh! He doesn't like the way this is going. I don't either.

Ali exacted the choral discipline with the lightest touch. Before trying out a demanding four-part harmony for the first time, she would bow and say 'Shall we?' or 'See you on the other side'. If anyone sang a false note she would thank them for improvising. She had something of Guillermo's diamond brilliance, but softened; where he would murmur: 'You know, you are not so very important' when a singer cringed at some blunder, Ali just reminded us that it really didn't matter. 'Be at peace,' she would say whenever we scrambled the rhythm, or forgot our parts halfway through the verse. We were amateurs, after all. If one of the parts got out of synch, she would stop them with a gesture, then her own strong voice would herd them safely in at the start of the next verse, her voice fading as theirs lifted. She was our shepherd, our sheepdog.

Ali had a dog of her own, Yoda, and when Yoda fell ill one summer term, and died on a Monday, she cancelled that Wednesday's class, then the next one. 'I find that I don't have a song in my heart,' she texted me. I emailed the group to tell them, and they sent condolences, even the ones who didn't get the message in time and turned up at the hall. Nobody thought that her reaction was excessive. She had made us that much of a unit.

Ali's throat hurt after Yoda died, and she mentioned tests and drugs. I always arrived early to put out the chairs and fill the water jugs, and she would tell me snippets about her life; how her throat was feeling, the anti-depressants she had been prescribed, the neighbour who was making her life difficult. I gathered that she lived alone, though she never said, and I winced at the strain of it. The group began to notice that she had less energy. All the parts of all those songs, filed in Ali's brain, almost nothing on paper, evaded her sometimes, and she would laugh too loudly, and frown, moving her lips. The numbers at each session began to drop. I could tell she was worried about the money, but when I tried to talk about charging more or moving to a cheaper venue, she evaded me. I wasn't really her friend, though I would have been glad to be. I put my hand on her arm once, when Yoda got his fatal diagnosis, and she stepped back. So I sent out the emails, and put out the chairs, and stood in the circle, and sang my part, and waited.

Yoda's anniversary came round this summer, and Ali's throat hurt again. I had the strongest feeling that she would not continue the group after the August break, but she said nothing, and I didn't like to ask. When I sent out the reminder email for the final meeting of the summer term, I headed it 'Swan Song', not thinking what that implied. But sure enough, Ali told me before the session, and the others during it, that she was taking time away from teaching. She needed a break. The group was curiously quiet. Knowing it was the last time, they lost cohesion: every singer for herself, and almost all the women insisted on taking the top part instead of sharing the lower ones. Kath and I, with more public spirit than competence, did our best to haul along the alto line, but it slipped from our grasp, and Ali had to leave the centre to stand with us. My voice is quite strong after years of practice, but there was not much sound there. My neck hurt, and Kath was clearing her throat too. At the end of that last lesson, leaving us, Ali said as usual, 'Be at peace'.

That was the last week of July. I've been thinking about Ali a lot since then, especially this last week, writing about singing and what it has meant to me. Steve and I are still in touch with some of the group, occasionally meeting them in Ali-less sessions with other leaders. We have been wondering if we could arrange our own workshop with Ali, just for one day, paying a fixed rate so she needn't worry about the numbers. Kath and some of the others were all for it. I was thinking I would make contact soon with Ali, and ask her if she felt up to it.

Then late last night, I got an email from Clare, the leader of another choir, a friend of Ali's who knew about our group.

'Terribly sad news..', it read. 'So sorry to tell you… at the weekend, in her home… took her own life'.

It is strange how you can be terribly shocked without being terribly surprised.

I had to send another email to Ali's choir, the first in four months, and all day long the replies have been coming back. 'I can hardly believe it'. Neither can I, except I also can. 'Poor Ali, she cared for us so much, so little for herself.' Yes. I think, now, that she was giving out far more than she actually had, and refusing to take anything back. 'She is an angel who has found her wings, but far too soon'. Not how I would have put it, but I hope that what she found, in death, was what she was looking for. 'She'd want us to keep singing'. True, probably. But I don't think that I have a song in my heart.

Ali has been leading groups in this area for twenty years. There will be hundreds of people mourning her today. It is strange that somebody can be so loved and valued, their face and voice so rich with light and depth, while their inner world is too monochrome and silent and solitary to sustain life.

I don't know to mourn this loss. I don't even have much idea, today, what I am mourning. Ali was a big person in my life, but not as big as this. I think it may take a long time. My life will go on, and will be about finding out. I don't know how Ali died. I hope it wasn't... anything that damaged her throat. My own throat might as well have been slashed in two. My song for Ali, today, is a growly, guttural groan.

Who's Your Friend?

ALI, BLESS HER dear heart, was never exactly my friend, but some of the people I met through my search for Help really were. Are. My psychotherapist self has a moment of uneasiness here, because psychotherapists becoming friends with their clients is mostly frowned upon in the profession, and I frown too. The relationship is too unequal during deep therapy, with enormous feelings projected on the therapist – feelings that belong really to mother, father, lover, their true self – for the two people involved, the two flawed, unique, ordinary people that make up the therapy dyad, to find a position of equal friendliness after the weekly intensity finishes. At least, I've never seen it work really well, though I've seen it attempted.

I can imagine that in theory problems could also emerge with osteopaths and so on making friends with clients, but I never experienced any. Our wedding photos show Venn-diagram-style overlaps of Help-related guests. That tableful of Elaine's patients included some that I'd originally met as professionals in other areas. Carollyn, the soprano who started out as my piano teacher and choir leader, and who sang during the signing of the register, was, through me, friends with Drew, the yoga teacher who followed

Miranda when I started working on Thursday evenings and had leave her class. Drew was a brilliant teacher and also a drummer, part of the jazz trio who played for us. Marianna was there too, a golden-hearted Austrian matriarch who personified my third attempt at Alexander Technique and my introduction (first time lucky, for once) to Qi Gong. She soon became my great friend and bridge opponent, partnering her daughter Juliette whose classic (not cranial) osteopathy was so valuable when I had my frozen shoulder. Marianna had been introduced by the homeopath recommended by Elaine… and so on.

By the time the wedding came round we were not seeing so much of Guillermo, who by then had moved away from South London. For over a year he had run a fabulous singing group in our home, integrating into our lives and those of our local acquaintances without becoming a friend in the sense of somebody you'd think of meeting for a pint. We sometimes finished the singing with a bottle of wine, and Guillermo would enjoy a glass, explaining as he took out his car keys, 'It does not affect me. I am from Argentina'. Had he downed the whole bottle, I probably would not have raised an eyebrow; somebody who has offered so much solid help is hard to criticise, even on those occasions when a protest might have been in order. I did not forget the fried egg.

All these friendships started organically, cautiously even. I can only recall one occasion when an overture came too soon from a professional, and I was quite disturbed by it. Trinny was my first Alexander Technique teacher, and I went to her looking for help with holding my head more steadily. When I mentioned my eye condition in the initial consultation, she looked quite excited.

'Really? I have a similar problem, only my night vision is poor and I see hallows round lamps.'

'Mm. I don't have anything like that. That sounds more like glaucoma. Anyway…'

'Glaucoma, you think?'

'I don't know. Haven't you seen an optician?'

'No. You're a doctor, you said?'

'A psychotherapist. Anyway…'

'Oh, I've been looking for some counselling since my partner died. Shall we do a swap?'

'Well… no. I just want some Alexander lessons. But I'm sorry about your partner. Was it long ago?'

She gulped. 'Saturday!'

Honestly, I'm not making it up. This conversation took place on a Tuesday. I could have told her she should take at least two weeks off, in fact I probably did, so deafening was her own emergency siren, louder by far than mine. In that initial session she eventually remembered who was consulting whom, but not before she'd invited me to her birthday party and insisted on lending me a book I didn't want to borrow, written by an old friend to whose life history she returned frequently during the lesson. I wish I could say that I never went back after that first session, but I did, several times, until the moment when I was lying on her couch and she picked up a full-length mirror to show me some distortion in my shoulders, and dropped it on top of me. Fortunately the mirror didn't shatter, but our uneasy alliance did. Definitely not wedding guest material.

Lest I began to sound like somebody whose mates are entirely selected from a directory of alternative therapies, I would like to add that I have other friends, acquired in the course of everyday life. Our relationships include all the usual things like enjoying each others' company, talking things over, helping each other out and so on, but my physiology's rather specific demands have more influence than I would like. My ability to have a varied social life is, for a basically able-bodied person, surprisingly limited. I'm always declining to go for a walk if it's slippery, or admitting that I had my eyes closed during a film because it was flickery, or refusing to go to the theatre unless I can sit in one of about ten seats, usually the most expensive, at the optimum angle from the stage. And I get terribly, terribly tired and dizzy just walking around looking at things, especially unfamiliar things, so fifteen minutes in an art gallery or a shopping centre sees me sinking on to a bench with my head in my hands. There are plenty of things I can and do enjoy doing in company – I'm a dab hand at eating and drinking, so long as the lighting is right and the venue accessible by train or foot - but I am always aware of an unwelcome choice between risking becoming so ill that the activity is curtailed anyway, or being upfront about my needs and cutting across those of the others. I know I am not the only person needing some kind of special consideration; far from it, especially as we all get older.

At the time of writing, the worst thing is my motion sickness. Apart from my day to day reluctance to get in a car or a bus, I offended two old friends recently by refusing invitations for birthday celebrations because I couldn't face the journey. One of them settled for her second-favourite venue thinking that I would prefer a flight to a ferry, but flying makes me ill too, and the drive from the airport was twisty, and it would be the hottest time of year with the sun lasering my dark glasses, and... No. Sorry. Really sorry. I've already got a flight booked for a holiday in the spring, and

I can't face two trips in one year. Really, really sorry. My neck has been awful recently. If you'd chosen somewhere in the UK… Oh alright, I'll shut up.

Details, details. I am describing my medical condition, my experiences, my conclusions about what worked and what didn't, in the hope of passing on something that in a general way will be useful to those undergoing all kinds of other conditions and experiences. In that spirit, just as I would recommend persevering with alternative therapies, I would recommend looking for a support group.

The support group I found, though not until my mid-thirties, was called the Nystagmus Action Group. 'NAG' for short, and the name was soon amended to 'Nystagmus Network' after an ophthalmologist observed that if we were trying to get professionals on side, we shouldn't threaten to nag them. Nystagmus Network, or NN.

NN did all kinds of useful things, and still does: improving understanding of nystagmus amongst medical and teaching professionals, sponsoring and taking part in research, putting people affected by nystagmus in touch with each other, and much more. I believe in its aims and I am one of many who have devoted aeons of free time to helping it flourish, but by far the best thing about it was simply being with other people who know what it's like.

My first encounter with NN was at an Open Day held in a North London hospital. I went on my own and there was the usual problem of finding the hospital from the tube, the signs positioned at unhelpful distances along the route, the disorientation in a small coppice beyond the station, and so on. Then the building itself; the confusion of neon-dazzled corridors. As I stood blinking, I heard voices ahead of me:

'Is that a turning up there, or just a dead end?'

'No idea!'

I followed the two young women who were laughing over their uncertainty, one hugging a small baby who laughed too, and I silently shared their triumph when it turned out that there *was* a turning, and that it led straight to the registration desk. What a great attitude, to walk the length of a corridor in a spirit of open curiosity, instead of sauntering to the end and turning back with deliberate carelessness when there was nothing there, like a snoozing cat pretending that it deliberately fell off the radiator.

I was enjoying myself already. Amongst all the buzz and busy-ness I felt absolutely unselfconscious, chatting to anyone I bumped into. I travelled home on the tube with one of the founder members and her son, and I enjoyed Vivien's friendly, detailed questions about my life and how I was managing. This was something that quickly became familiar in that group: the sheer good will pouring from the parents of children with nystagmus towards the adults. They wanted us to succeed and be happy so that their children would, and they valued any positive example we were able to set. At that first meeting I heard a little girl ask:

'How will I get to places when I'm grown up and can't drive?'

Her mum gestured to one of the committee, a tall, smiling young man with a job on a national newspaper, and told her,

'You'll get on a bus, like Big John.'

John and the little one beamed.

It was lovely to feel normal. I joined the committee, and when at the first meeting I attended everyone picked up their agendas, I was astonished to see them position the paper right in front of their eyes. How weird! But of course, that was what I did. Once, our usual venue being unavailable, a meeting was held in somebody's flat in the Barbican, and there was only minimal, sympathetic comment when one of the members totally failed to find the place, and had to go home after an hour of searching. It was just one of those things.

It was just one of those things, nothing odd at all. I was able, for the first time, to share the confusion I once experienced trying to post a letter in an unfamiliar street. Through crowds of pedestrians I glimpsed a post box some way ahead, but obviously further than it seemed, because I took ages reaching it. I broke into a trot finally, only to find that the post box was actually a woman wearing a red coat and a black beret. The missing detail, you see.

My new nystagmic friends knew just what I meant, and recounted howlers of their own. Nystagmus, being really a symptom of a neurological problem and not a condition in itself, can affect people very differently, but the difficulties with judging distance and movement are common, and also extreme fatigue when looking at things, especially confusing ones like supermarket shelves or close type. There was much useful advice on offer. 'Try turning the page on its side,' somebody said when I was staring dizzily at a list of names, trying to work out whether 'Collman' had one or two Ls. And yes, when I turned the page ninety degrees, there were the two Ls, now lying separately one above the other where before they had woozed and merged.

NN was entirely run by volunteers when I joined, but a few years later funding was found for a part-time employee, and I had the honour of being the first to hold that role. As Information and Development Officer I was first in line picking up the phone to potential members, some of them shell-shocked parents of recently diagnosed babies. Some had been given misleading information by the hospital and expected terrible things, others had no information at all.

'Will she go to school like normal children?'

'Will he be able to work?'

'Will she drive a car?'

'Yes.'

'Almost certainly yes.'

'Probably not, but a few people with nystagmus can.'

The relief of just speaking to a normal sounding, reasonably cheerful adult with a condition like their child's brought many of the parents to tears.

Some desperate callers fired personal questions which I never resented, but found harder to answer.

'Did you do OK at school?'

'Yes, I did pretty well.'

'Have you got a degree?'

'Yes.'

'What degree?'

'French and Philosophy.'

'I mean, what class?'

'Um – a 2:2' (sorry).

'Do you read for pleasure? My husband and I love reading…' (sob).

'Yes, I love reading. Most of us do, in NN.'

'Oh, good. Are you married?'

'Um, no.'

'Are you not married because you have nystagmus?'

'Well…'

Where is that controlled trial when you need it? Would I have fallen in love and got married earlier, perhaps had babies of my own, if not for that scrap of neurological damage? How on earth can I know? Perhaps it is a sad question for anybody: what would I have been if this, if not that. All I could say, truthfully, to the questioning parents, was even with the actual this and that, I was very glad to be here.

DIY

I AM A seasoned psychotherapist nowadays, no longer a systems analyst or an information officer or a researcher, though I consider myself lucky to have had this portfolio of professions to hand, some of which have run concurrently with my psychotherapist practice. Belated apologies to Annie for being so suspicious on that score.

I have a theory that the majority of people who train as psychotherapists or counsellors, do so because they are looking for something for themselves, not because they think that talking therapies offer an attractive, or even a feasible, career path. I am so interested in this idea, which is by no means unique to me, that a few years ago I carried out my own research on the subject, conducting semi-structured interviews and posting online surveys, then analysing the results and writing it all up. It was published by Karnac as a chapter in a book that included work by the then prestigious Camila Batmanghelidjh, who unfortunately was discredited just after it was published (nothing to do with the book). I am not sure if anybody ever bought a copy, let alone read it. It still has no reviews on Amazon.

I enjoyed the research process, using the skills I'd acquired the previous year while writing my MA dissertation. I sense the pricking up of ears, no doubt those of that parent on the long ago Nystagmus Network phone line.

'What class of MA?'

'Distinction.'

'Really? Then why didn't you do better in your first degree? Was it because…'

Well, it might have been. A part-time, dissertation only MA is less taxing on the eyes than all the paraphernalia of lectures and handwritten notes and unreadable OHPs and the other horrors that go with a full-time first degree. Maybe one of those other Mes in the trial got a 2:1; perhaps, if imagination runs wild, even a First, and these were the days when Firsts were as rare as dodos. And here Imagination runs slap into the memory of Tim in the Civil Service, packing his Ursula Le Guins into the filing cabinet next to the biking magazines, pulling on his leather jacket and remarking,

'If I'd gone to university, I've have got a First. But I didn't want to go.'

A dubious silence from me, a snort from Phil. This is the problem with controlled trials, if imaginary. The results of my research into why people train as talking therapists had the advantage of being based on the present universe. I focused on people who were paying for their own training, not those trained up as part of an existing job. And the amounts they paid! – tens of thousands for course fees and supervision fees and personal therapy during the training, to say nothing of the incidental expenses and lost earnings in their day jobs, and the emotional wear and tear. The sums are clearly beyond the reach of folk with very modest resources, but the people I interviewed were not rich either, and mostly relied on loans or legacies plus the earnings of their spouses.

And, I asked, how many of these would be therapists worked out, before committing to this outlay, how soon they would cover the cost of the training, let alone make any kind of living? Hardly any. In fact, how many succeeded in finding any therapy work at all after qualifying, paid work that is, not the endless 'placements' offered by charities, colleges, even the NHS? About half. It follows that many people were gaining these vocational qualifications for other reasons, their own reasons.

I was one of them. I was in my thirties; my mother had died; I was working as a systems analyst/programmer in the IT department of a children's charity, and just about managing the screen work, provided I took things quietly in the evenings. I understood that it was gradually doing my head in and that I needed a career change, but how many jobs of which I was capable did not involve sitting at a computer for hours on end, or driving a car? Well – psychotherapy, of course.

I was a believer, in a cautious sort of way. My time with Jennifer especially, and to some extent with Robin, had given me confidence that it could work. I even heard later that Madeleine in her heyday had helped some people. I had been miserable when Jennifer told me she was leaving London so we would have to stop – 'and I'm sorry, because I know it is too soon for you'. Feelings in therapy can run high, and I felt pretty much the same as the afternoon I got home from the sweet shop, aged nine, to find the door locked and a note saying that my parents had gone out for a couple of hours. Jennifer gave me a notice period, most of which I spent groaning: 'And now that you're moving to Milton Keynes...' with Jennifer interrupting: 'It's St Albans. Don't go making it worse than it is.' Then the minute hand of her clock would tick to '50' and it would be time to leave, emphasising the stinginess of the therapy hour and indeed the whole therapy process. Sometimes I hated it more than I loved it.

So it was awful being abandoned by Jennifer, but if she had stayed in London I might never have found James, and my life would have been quite different. As well as being an ordained priest, apparently, he practised something called Body Psychotherapy. I had never heard of it, and it sounded like a contradiction in terms, but a fairly sane looking woman I knew from work claimed that well as sorting out her failing marriage, James had cured her of all kinds of physical maladies, and the thought of that happening for me was irresistible.

So I made an appointment and turned up at his swanky flat in West London. It was a far cry from Madeleine's scout hut or Robin's wardrobe or Jennifer's tiny studio. The wide hall was carpeted with kilim rugs and lined with abstract paintings and scattered with pieces of modern sculpture. In his dark blue office I sat in a comfortable chair and said a bit about my life in general and a great deal about my feelings for Jennifer, which I found rather irritating. I was beginning to suspect, even at this early stage, that the therapy world was largely self-referential, and my study for the Karnac book supported this theory, suggesting that on the whole it is therapists who like to receive therapy.

James was a cuddly man with a white beard and a cheerful laugh, and I felt quite ready to confide in him, though I was distracted by the bookshelf behind his head, which housed what looked like a plastic Santa clutching a parcel and propping up a shopping list. In June! What did this mean? Did James suffer from some seasonal compulsive disorder which impelled him to buy his Christmas presents in the summer? I never found out.

Anyway, the body psychotherapy was a revelation. I had lain on plenty of couches in my time, but this one was a place to notice, and voice, all the feelings they held. The ancient, doctor-induced terrors, the vulnerability, the relief at having my head supported, the sensual pleasure of James's thigh against my arm, the regressive rush of longing when he held my hand silently for five minutes then said, 'How was that?' I loved James; I adored him. I'd have married him, during the session itself if he wouldn't make time for me outside. He was an ordained minister after all, maybe he could marry *us* as well as marrying *me*.

So it came as a shock when a few weeks into the therapy, James told me he was emigrating to Australia. *What?*

'I've unexpectedly been offered a job', he blustered, and I thought:

'LIAR! Why would somebody in Australia offer you a job, unprovoked?'

Further investigations via the woman who recommended him, revealed that he had a partner already living in Sydney, a man who, for many months, had been sending him details of vacancies. James had always been planning to dump me.

I seethed, but still I loved him, and still some inner voice whispered that we could be happy together. What if he seemed unattainable because of being my therapist, and in a relationship, and gay, and moving to the other side of the world? Love could find a way... Six sessions later he left the country, and I recovered quite quickly, perhaps because there was so little reality in all that passion. But the body psychotherapy seed was sown, and grew strong. I found out where James did his training and applied on my own account. I vaguely hoped that by offering this powerful work I would be able to help other people and make some kind of new career for myself, but I suspect that I was mainly trying to help myself by becoming, in some way, my own inner James, my own inner Jennifer; my very own James-and-Jennifer, who this time would not leave me.

I was still working full-time for the charity when I started my training, and I gawp now at the timetable that I endured for the first two years. The course was designed to fit around full-time 9-5 working days – why? did only super-heroes apply? In term time, my Tuesdays and Thursdays consisted of eight hours at the computer followed by ninety minutes of rush hour between South East and North West London, then three hours of intense and often emotional concentration, then eighty minutes back home, if I was lucky. Being lucky meant catching the 10:08 from Ealing Broadway, but if the session ran over and I got a later train, the connections didn't work so well and I wasn't home much before midnight.

The journey itself was terrifying, with much standing on deserted platforms and at dark bus stops that pulsed with London life. Loud young men in leather jackets. Seedy old men breathing beer. Horrible. I lived on my own at that time, and I would slam my front door behind me, relishing the sense of my own space wrapping itself around me, but still humming with adrenaline, so that sleep was a long time coming. Then an early start in the morning, and more computers. Oh, and there were weekend classes too, some weeks on both Saturday and Sunday. At the end of the second year I gave up my IT job and started part-time in the Nystagmus Network role, so the week became a bit easier. It was worth the drop in income.

I paid for my training out of money my mother left me, and it is only now, writing this, that I reflect how appalled she would be to find that I spent her careful savings, much of it inherited from her own mother, in such a stressful way. There is something brutal about inheritance. You hand over your loved one, perhaps a mother you are only just starting to truly value, and in return Death passes you a suitcase of used notes. You lug it to your bank, and there your ill-gotten gains fester, bubbling with interest, waiting for you to come up with some object or project that is worth the exchange. Oh, I know I sound privileged, being able to leave the money there for years, waiting to find an appropriate, or at least bearable, use for it. Many people would have immediate needs, for better housing or better food, or support for their dependents. But I had no dependents, I was in work, and I'd always heeded Mum's advice to live within my income. So the inheritance was there waiting, and the prospect of acquiring my own inner James-and-Jennifer, my own inner good parent in fact, finally seemed like a fair exchange.

My poor mother, who after I moved to London used to insist on giving me taxi money whenever she dropped me off at the station, would have quailed at all that late-night trudging, occasionally running, when things got nasty, through the London streets and underground.

Mum might not have been that impressed by the course either. Even I only liked parts of it. For months I was baffled by a module called 'Body and Energy'. What on earth was this 'energy' they were speaking of? It might have made more sense if I had not been in a state of chronic exhaustion. My eyelids drooped the moment I sat down, and when we moved from the theory with which our sessions always started to the practical work, I would discover that I had taken in a fraction of what was said. Only the memory of James, James and how he had made me feel, prevented me from giving up. James had definitely been doing *something*, and I wanted to do it too.

Sure enough, aided by hands on experience in the 'Biodynamic Massage' module, light eventually dawned. I remember the first time it happened, working with a woman called Caroline who later became a great friend, but at that moment was a near stranger with whom I was not on particularly good terms. As instructed, I placed my right hand on Caroline's hip and my left hand on her knee, and tried to visualise this 'energy' thing moving between my hands. And suddenly I felt it! A deep, gentle pulsing, looping slowly but strongly through Caroline's flesh, into my left hand, out again, back into my right hand, round and round. Even when the energy wasn't 'in' either of my hands, I could somehow track its position in Caroline's thigh. We were told to leave the left hand on the knee and move the right hand to the ankle. A moment's pause, and the looping began again, faintly at first, then stronger. Caroline's leg gave a small, comfortable stretch and I saw colour come into her cheeks. At the end, we thanked each other with a genuine smile.

There were many other modules as the four years went on, more than I can remember now. There was some kind of encounter group in which we were supposed to interact with each other and discuss how it felt. I have never liked talk for the sake of it, and I was often bored in that one, or irritated, as well as tired. Then there were endless hours of 'triangles' in which talking therapy was practised, each triangle made up of a client, therapist and observer. I hated being observed as either client or therapist, even though I recognised that we needed both practice and feedback. When I eventually got to the point of being qualified, and seeing clients one-to-one in a private room, the relief of finally being unobserved overcame much of my initial nervousness.

But there was a long and hard way to go before that point. It is taxing, spending time with people struggling with enormous personal issues, and many of us were in that position. If therapy is provocative, therapy trainings are even more so, and the bodywork, with its invitation to vulnerability, particularly so. Themes recurred. I remember sitting in a random group of six students, and three of them turned out to have a dead sibling. Incest and sexual abuse left their mark all over the place, and also trauma following medical treatment. I was still some way from registering properly that my eye surgery had been traumatic, but I could not ignore the recurring signposts. On one occasion there was talk about somebody waking up during an operation, and I literally froze, I was unable to move a muscle, until the tutor noticed and managed to talk me back to mobility. Another time, as client, I began to shake violently when describing a series of attacks that was baffling the police in the area where I lived. The object of the attack, always an old person living alone, and often bedridden, would be woken in the night by a torch shining in their face, whereupon the perpetrator, who had gained entry by picking a lock or removing a window, cutting their phone cable as he mounted the stairs, would sexually assault his victim and escape with their valuables. The thoroughness and efficiency of these attacks made them particularly horrible, but the victims were more than twice my age, and my therapist puzzled over my visceral identification with them. Then he said, 'Actually, it is not the thought of the break-in or the assault or the robbery that seems to be bothering you, but the idea of a torch shining in your eyes.'

I don't know whether I woke up during one of my operations, but it is possible. Joshua Lang, quoted in The Atlantic journal, says that of every thousand patients undergoing surgery, between one and two wake up during the operation. The writer is quick to assure us that most of them are awake for as little as five minutes, and 'not all of them experienced pain... only about eighteen per cent'. How many people have surgery each year, worldwide? How many people is eighteen per cent of one or two in a thousand of that number? A lot of people. A lot. Maybe I was one of them. Oh, and five minutes in those circumstances may not pass as quickly to the patient as to the surgeon. I don't understand how these figures can be quoted so calmly.

One thing the training did for me, was to normalise my dreaded 'sensitivity'. I was not the only one freezing and trembling at the mention of certain subjects. Plenty of snowflakes there, a perfect snowstorm some days. I did get much more 'in touch', as we body psychotherapists say, with my own body, which led to me feeling more 'at home' in it, as we also say. And I gained the basics for a career which I have practised with consistent interest and frequent joy for two decades, full of satisfying contact with other human beings. But did the training provide that inner James-and-Jennifer that I longed for? No. Did it help me understand myself better? A bit, but not as much as my personal therapy. The people who really made a difference came later: Elaine, and Miranda, and Drew, and certain spiritual teachings, and, of course, Guillermo. The training paved the way for some of that. I would not have received so much from cranial-sacral work, or osteopathy, if I had not learnt to feel energy. But those were the people who really helped.

Hmm. So am I one of the small number of therapists in my survey who trained mostly for the career prospects, not the personal development? No! I was in it for the personal stuff, though in the end I got more from practising than training. I wonder whether my mother, wherever she is, considers it money well spent.

In Practice

So FOR A good part of the time I was looking for help, trying out hypnotherapists and osteopaths and so on, and learning to sing, I was a trainee or practising body psychotherapist myself. I say this not just to clarify timelines for my reader, but to remind myself that this was the case. I felt so very straightforwardly a client, somebody with a problem she could not solve herself seeking professional help, not at all like somebody with inside information. No, that isn't quite true. When I saw Trinny, the Alexander Technique teacher with the undiagnosed glaucoma and the recently deceased partner, a siren went off in my head, but that was to do with boundaries, not about the way she worked at her own modality. As far as the actual sessions went, she was the teacher and I the student.

So did it help me, going through all that training, and then working with my own clients? Yes, in some ways. When my work helps a client, it helps me too. This happens in a very direct way with massage; a session that clears and settles a client's energy, clears and settles mine too. More generally, if somebody's life becomes more comfortable/satisfying/ joyful/tolerable from working with me, that adds pleasure and meaning to my life too. And I think it often helps to really immerse yourself in another person's mental world, when things are getting a bit sticky in your own head.

For somebody like me, whose discomfort expresses itself in very bodily ways, it is helpful just to be reminded of the way physical pain can be a sign of mental torment. Guillermo would agree there. In the early days of singing with him, I was plagued by a catch in my voice that I would try to counteract by coughing or clearing my throat ('Don't do that! That is a violent thing to do!'). It felt like phlegm, but Guillermo was sure that the catch or tremor came from some misalignment of my upper body and/or from my emotional state, which with my body psychotherapy hat on I think are two sides of the same coin. 'You are lucky,' he would say, 'that your voice expresses so clearly how you are. It will be a guide for you.' Yup, I was a finely-tuned instrument alright.

Theories abound about the relationship between physical malaise and spiritual/psychic distress, and most of these theories are too glib for my taste. 'Cancer/dementia/heart disease is the result of suppressed anger', says one theory, and I can only think that it might be in some cases, but in general these serious illnesses are at least as likely to be due to environmental/lifestyle/genetic factors. It puts such a burden on a suffering person to suggest, even obliquely, that their illness is 'their own fault'. I've heard it said that even things apparently beyond a person's control, like being a passenger in a train crash, only happen if the person in some way wants it to. I don't believe that for a moment. A train crash is a train crash.

But I do believe that emotional distress can make its home in the body, and that listening to what the body has to say can be the first step to feeling better. I can't use examples from my client work, but I can mention non-clients with whom I occasionally do bits of bodywork.

One example: a friend arrived for a weekend visit with a very painful hip. She did not remember ever having a similar problem before, and had no idea what caused it; she had been 'just standing around' that morning when it started hurting. As it was a Friday evening and there was no chance of finding any other treatment, I did a bit of energy work and gentle massage on her hip, but it didn't make much difference, except to relax the muscles around the painful spot. So I asked her to notice whether the pain changed at all while I named a few things that she'd said were going on in her life. Her intrusive new neighbour? No. Her husband's decision to take early retirement? No. Her daughter? Ouch! And then she remembered how the pain started. She had been standing in the shopping centre, leaning against the railings above a staircase, when she caught a glimpse of her daughter's distinctive white coat and blonde curly hair disappearing into a shop that offered cosmetic surgery and botox. This young woman had a history of over-using such treatments to the detriment of her health, and of over-spending in general, but she had assured her mother that she had put a stop to all that. When my friend stepped away from the railings, her hip seemed to give way, and she had been hobbling ever since. So how *was* she feeling about her daughter? 'I'm just scared,' she said, and sobbed briefly. 'I don't know if she tells me the truth, and I don't know what sort of future she'll have if she carries on like this, and I don't know how to help her'.

My friend never found out whether it actually was her daughter going into that beauty parlour that day, or just somebody who looked similar from the back, but that was not the point. As far as her body was concerned, it had happened. After the treatment she was no closer than before to being able to sort out her daughter's life, but paying attention to her hip pain, then allowing herself to feel and express the feelings that set it off, provided relief. The pain disappeared, and by the time she left on Sunday evening, it had not come back.

Those fifteen minutes of impromptu therapy helped my friend, and they helped me too, partly because helping one's friend is a pleasure, and also by reminding me, yet again, that at least some of my own joint pain and dizziness and so on, is likely to be an expression of emotional discomfort. I don't think that all of it is. I really am holding my head in an unsustainable position, and that is bound to put my muscular-skeletal system out. I really do have 'a bit of brain damage', as that doctor put it, and my eyes really do have an involuntary wobble. I really have repeatedly pulled and twisted parts of my body in the past, making them more susceptible to future injuries. It would be surprising to attain perfect ease in these circumstances.

Having recognised all this, it may still be true that some or all of a particular pain on a particular occasion has an emotional element, and sometimes I do a bit of body psychotherapy on myself. Anybody can try it. It might go like this:

You're sitting at your computer when you realise that your neck is stiff. Check that out: is 'stiff' the best word? No! There's a sharp pain too. Ouch.

Ask yourself a typical body psychotherapy question: 'What would that pain in your neck be saying, if it could speak?' Well, 'pain in the neck' says a lot already. Who or what has been a pain in the neck recently? You may get an answer at once, but if not, keep going.

'If something physical was causing that pain, what would it be? Is it like being stabbed with a knife maybe, or like being twisted?'

Take a bit of time to feel what is going on (this will help on its own, if nothing else does. Our bodies like our own attention best of all.) Well – unlikely as it may seem, the feeling in your neck might be of a sort that is caused by somebody dragging your head backwards. And now you notice a related twinge in your shoulder blade, almost as if somebody was twisting your arm.

Back to the first question: 'who or what…?' Perhaps your attention is drawn to the email icon on the screen in front of you, and you start thinking about a message from a colleague who has emailed you at home, at the weekend, asking you to do something that isn't your job and that they could perfectly well do themselves. Talk about neurotically entitled! Do they imagine that you are their PA? Just the sort of way your dad might have treated you, pompous patriarchal git that he was!

Perhaps there's a fizzing in your oesophagus, as if something was trying to get out. What would you like to say to your colleague and/or your dad, without editing or softening your words? The immediate response to this kind of question, by the way, rarely turns out to be something it would be politic to say in real life, especially to somebody you need to get on with. But now, on your own, give it some welly. Try a few expletives. Would that be more satisfying at louder volume? Would that twisted arm enjoy throwing a punch? Try it!

You don't have to smash the place up, but it can make a big difference to allow these trapped sounds and movements to express themselves, even in a small way. Check in with your neck and shoulder. Do they need more? When they feel better, then job done, until the next time.

Talking of God...

ALI WAS A Christian, it seems from the social media snippets, or at least she played in a Christian band for a while. I wouldn't have guessed from talking to her. The only time she mentioned religion was to say how much she hated Christmas. She taught us gospel songs, but they stand on their own musical merits.

Whatever Ali's faith was, and however much it may have helped her along the way, evidence shows that it didn't, in the end, make her life worth living. That raises a question for me: how much has my own faith or spiritual practice helped when it came to my neurological blip and my traumatised response to the medical treatment? Has there been any kind of healing along those lines?

I count myself lucky that I have always, since I can remember, had a sense of God. I say 'God' for want of a better word; an earlier draft of this very chapter included a long-winded attempt to find an alternative, but by definition there can be no adequate definition that fits into human language. I mean by God some kind of energy that includes but is bigger than the whole natural world, including humankind, and that will continue after we are gone, which with the current environmental crisis may not be very far ahead. I'll use the traditional pronoun 'he' because 'she' or 'it' or 'them' would be no more or less adequate.

As my mother complained, I did not come from a family of believers, being brought up in house without a Bible, let alone any other religious text, where such matters were not discussed, even as a palliative for the sadness of life. No 'Granny's gone to be an Angel in Heaven' for us. I asked Mum what death was, the first time I heard the word in infant school, and my question seemed to surprise her, as though the answer was obvious.

'People aren't here forever, you know. At some point, usually when they're old, they sort of go away.'

'Go away how, where?'

'Well, they fall over, and their body goes cold and stiff, and then it is buried in the ground'.

'Oh. Right...'

Perhaps in search of something less bald, I read the Gideon New Testament provided by the school in my bedroom of an evening while my peers congregated in the park, smoking or testing the narcotic powers of cough syrup. Some bits I skipped– the Acts of the Apostles were scrappy and unconvincing – but others, especially the Sermon on the Mount, were as piquant as my favourite meal of kippers and meringues, to be savoured and lingered over. I took to prayer early and easily, discussing what was going on with God and asking sometimes for interventions, but continuing unfazed if they were not forthcoming.

Did any of this prayer and Bible reading, this sense of God being around, help with the neurology/trauma stuff? A bit, I think. It made me feel safer and more balanced, gave me a sense of something bigger and more reliable standing behind me, into whose arms I could fall back, like in that game of Trust. Having said that, I don't remember God being around after the eye operations, though perhaps I would not remember, being so young. I prayed for Mum while she was ill, but always with a sense that her time was short, and that 'sort of going away' was on the cards.

It is a gloomy possibility that when the chips are down, my faith will no help to me, especially if my body is very sick. I never gave God a thought during the post lumbar puncture weeks, even though I felt so ill that I was close to wishing for death. I gave myself a month, at one point, to feel better before pursuing that option. Life in so much physical pain, neither ears nor eyes operational, unable to raise my head from my pillow, was not worth living; it was hardly life at all.

Perhaps that is how Ali felt. Mental pain is just as bad as physical, and can have the same effect of wiping out other things, including the knowledge that one is loved and will be missed. Just as I forgot to brush my teeth during that time, forgot that such a thing as a toothbrush existed, I forgot to reach out for God.

I was aware from a fairly young age that faith was something best pursued in community, but I experienced in looking for such a community, similar problems to when I was looking for alternative therapies. As a teenager I joined a Baptist church and youth group, where I enjoyed singing the hymns even though I was convinced at that point that I was tone deaf (I see Ali and Guillermo roll their eyes at the detrimental effects of school singing lessons). Occasionally I got something from the sermons, but my hopes for Christian companionship amongst the Youth were thwarted by their astonishing enthusiasm for table tennis, which I lost every time because the ping pong ball disappeared as soon my opponent hit it. Foiled again by that scrap of damaged brain tissue.

At university I extended my search to a Methodist church, but that was not a success either. I still hoped that somebody in church would speak or act or even preach with the kippers-and-meringues exquisiteness of the Sermon on the Mount, but the people there just seemed very dull, much duller than people at University or even my family, and not always as generous or as kind. I'll never forget a Sunday in my first year, when I was hugely enjoying learning to play Bridge. We stopped earlier than we would have liked in order to go to the evening service, I and the friends I was playing with: a post-grad called Andrew, who had learnt Bridge at Oxford and was brilliant, my friend Janette who was about my level, and another girl called Janet who completely failed to grasp the rules, but with heavy prompting made an adequate fourth. After the service, the minister came over to wish us good evening and ask what we'd been doing that day. When we told him, he frowned.

'What's this? You've been playing games of chance, on a Sunday?'

'Games of chance? Oh no,' said Andrew, then, 'Well, Janet was.'

I never went back to that church. Andrew's wit and our joint pleasure in the game seemed to have more of God in them than that stodgy, stingy, nit-picking attitude. I should say a word here for Bridge, if played in the right company, which means people whom you like anyway, and who give each hand their complete attention without much caring who wins. It is convivial and absorbing and gives your brain a work-out in a rather similar way to singing. Good bridge can definitely help with gloom. I'd suggest avoiding bridge *clubs* unless you are very experienced, and very fast, and have nerves of steel. They can be bloody.

So my early church going experiences were not the best, but my quiet internal connection to God continued: a dropping down, from time to time, into a deep place of love and safety and truth. It is so hard to describe, and most likely quite boring for my reader. Personally I don't find much literature or even poetry about God all that engaging. Music does the job better. Rutter's 'Deep peace of the running wave to you' – now we're talking.

As usual for me, it was third time lucky, with a small Anglican church, 'low' and on the evangelical side, which stood in the South London street to which I moved after university. The church had no vicar, and was run by an ancient couple of ex-missionaries, Roy and Dora, who smiled on all they encountered with a kind of effortless humility that is only imitated at their peril by those whose natures lack it. Roy and Dora were backed up by a team of young people, around my own age, scattered in shared houses; my lawyer flatmate was one of them. Another, by coincidence, was the very person who had interviewed me for my charity fundraising job. The world of London was cosier than I'd expected, and God, to my delight, was an everyday subject of conversation in that little area. I can't remember now what was said, but the New Testament message of good news and community was acted out in everyday life. We were always cooking each other meals and helping out in practical ways, and the musical ones got together to practise wonderful songs for the services, and we found ways to help anyone who came to the church, including various homeless people and a young man who lived for over a year on various sofas then departed with some of our possessions, but nobody got cross. Somebody who lost a favourite watch, just said: 'Oh! I wish he'd just told us the truth'. I loved it there.

The only thing I disliked about being an evangelical Christian was having to evangelise, but I did it anyway, because I really believed that people were at risk of going to hell. I worried about this, at times, in the way that I now worry, at times, about climate change. It was many years before I realised that most of my co-evangelicals didn't believe anything of the sort, not really, even if they thought they did. They would surely have looked less cheerful if seriously facing the prospect of their friends and neighbours heading to hell. This thought bothered me only occasionally during my time in that church, but intensified at Bible College, especially with Mum not being a believer herself. Sometimes I tried to calculate what percentage of human beings would (according to evangelical principles) be saved. A fraction of one per cent, it must be, yet God kept wilfully creating more, apparently on the off-chance that a few of them would hear the Good News and repent.

My identity as an evangelical Christian was never the same after that, sickened as I was by a divine system that could sanction this eternal carnage. I went right off the idea of working overseas with people who had not heard the 'good' news. Instead I returned to my London church after the Bible course, but that wasn't the same either; my old friends had moved on too, but in different directions from me. I used to be an unofficial lay preacher, but there was less and less that I could truthfully say. Eventually I moved house a few miles away, and stopped attending.

Later on, when I told Jennifer all this, she remarked that whole belief systems can be discarded surprisingly quickly. I did not lose my sense of God, but my connection to him was stretched to the limit for some years. Either he was sulking, or I was. It was probably me, because there were times, like when my dad died, that something pinged back and I insisted on a religious funeral with those wonderful words 'now we commit his body to the ground, ashes to ashes, dust to dust'. Nothing else would do. I occasionally went back to the South London church and was kindly received by my old friends, but Roy and Dora had retired to Hastings and been replaced by a vicar, a vicar who seemed to think he was in charge, and who had no idea of the part I used to play there. With his robe and his collar and his sonorous voice, he laid a veil of churchliness over the old freedoms.

But I missed going to church, and gradually began to take my spiritual custom elsewhere. Indeed, I became what the evangelicals would call 'woolly', dabbling in Buddhist meditation and finding there the old sense of falling back into the arms of something huge and true. Buddhism also offered, in the Loving Kindness meditation, a shortcut to peaceful acceptance of the difficult people in my life, myself included. I began to appreciate more and more the benefits of accepting things as they are. Life really sucks sometimes, and it can feel better to sink to rock bottom and rest there, rather than fighting the current. To use a different analogy, a crisis is like being swept out to sea by a freak wave. Most people won't be strong enough to swim back to shore against the tide, so the trick is to breathe as well as possible, move your limbs enough to stay afloat, and go with the flow. Either you'll be swept back to shore or somebody will notice and send help. Safety is not guaranteed, but those are your best options.

Miranda enhanced my spiritual search, and I went to

all kinds of group activities arranged by her, where we lay on silk rugs and evoked the Archangel Michael or opened our spiritual portals to connect to various stars. Sometimes we sat round her huge, beautiful wax candles and took it in turns to draw a card from a pack decorated with unicorns, peering at messages which it was too dark to read accurately. If Miranda didn't like her message, she had a habit of returning it and choosing another. I felt that I was doing the same thing with my spirituality, picking and discarding until something felt right.

But did it help? Yes, I think that being a part of almost any spiritual community can help with almost anything so long as – what can I say – so long as the Spirit moves freely? All these phrases are so loaded. You have to feel at home, but I don't think it is a good idea to look too hard for a 'like-minded' group where a wish to toe the party line can get in the way of discovery. Miranda and I are unlike-minded in some ways, but like enough to nurture each other spiritually. More important for a group is whether its members are heading, or at least trying to head, in approximately the same direction.

I have found my second spiritual home now in Cumbria, at the Quakers. We are a small group from different backgrounds, and we don't necessarily think the same about God or anything else, but we are all looking, as Quakers say, for the Light. Meetings are mostly silent; we sit in a circle and ask for Light on our own situations, and other people's, and the world's, and the fact of doing it all together makes it more powerful. After an hour we shake hands and have a cup of tea and a chat, and that's it. We call each other Friends.

We call each other Friends, and being friendly is central:

'lifting one another up with a tender hand,' as Quaker Faith and Practice puts it. Listening to other people – all other people – is also central: 'Listen twice, speak once'. It feels like home to me, in a way which no church has done except that one in South London, but it is not perfect. Being a Friend doesn't guarantee that you always listen, or even that you are always friendly. And some take the quiet contemplation thing too far. An actor in a Quaker theatre company complained that for a comic play with an element of slapstick, some Friends in the front row arranged themselves with bowed heads and closed eyes, so that the company was left, in effect, performing to thin air.

Life is never perfect, and neither is anyone or anything in it. I remember in my Nystagmus Network days meeting a few guide dogs, and being naively astonished by some of their antics. One man arrived late for a meeting complaining that his dog, who supposedly knew the route, got distracted by a woman with sausages in her shopping basket, and followed her home instead. When I expressed my outrage at this lack of professionalism, the owner said, 'They're only dogs, you know.' It's the same with Quakers. We're only people.

Here's a funny thing. The majority of Friends at my Meeting, though younger than me, turn out to be dealing with some chronic physical problem. A rare autoimmune disease, or early arthritis, or whatever. One woman told me that if the sunshine from the window lingered on the back of her head for too long, she went temporarily blind – just the sort of thing that might happen to me. So we all have that in common, and we laugh about it and call ourselves 'the old crocks', though our average age is decades younger than some of the other local meetings. That helps. Some weeks I am the only one feeling robust enough to move around the chairs. I do enjoy being the able-bodied one. That helps too.

Back On The Hoarse

YESTERDAY STEVE AND I went to the drop-in choir run by Clare, the singing teacher who let me know about Ali dying. My voice seemed to have died with her; I hadn't managed so much as a hum since I heard the news, though Ali's songs continued to buzz in my head like trapped insects. 'This pretty planet, Spinning in space…' 'Oh Mother carry me, Your child I will always be…' It was horrible to experience the shattering of sound and meaning before it even reached my throat. I have only been singing for ten years, but it seems to be essential now. How strange for Ali to be the one who took that away.

We went to Clare's choir largely because she'd emailed to say that they would sing something in Ali's memory, which might be the closest we would ever get to attending a funeral. Apparently her family want to be left to mourn in their own way, and the community musicians who loved Ali and who would have otherwise have kept on spreading the word, have been respecting this. The tributes from her musical colleagues, when read more closely, indicate long-term mental health problems. At some point a coroner's report will go online, and I have to confess that I will be looking out for it.

So yesterday morning Steve and I got the early bus to an unfamiliar town hall, where we were greeted by some of our old group. Hugs were exchanged and we sat down in the circle, which was larger than anything Ali ever achieved in our own town hall. The numbers in our sessions were rarely high enough to cover costs and make a reasonable profit. Each week my stomach would rock as I counted the punters in, while Ali went quiet and fixed her eyes on the little blue cash box.

But here all was peace and plenty, and Clare stood in the centre of three rows of chairs, all occupied, while she read out, with barely a wobble, a tribute of which I heard about one word in five. Then we sang a song that Ali used to finish her sessions with: 'Shalom, my friend.' Some people sang it, anyway. Scattered amongst the rows were several bowed heads, and tears poured into my own hands, right down my sleeves, making my elbows wet and waterlogging my spare tissues. 'Till we meet again, till we meet again…' oh, Ali. We sang that to finish our very last meeting. I could see her there, in the centre, hands raised, drinking it in, smiling when she caught my eye. Smiling bravely, I think now.

What helps with grief? As most of us know, nothing helps much at first. Most of us know that crying can provide some relief, as can talking about the person you lost. It can help to understand exactly what you are grieving for, which may not be immediately obvious. Grief implies a large helping of longing, to see the person again, to hear them, to know they are OK; but there is usually more. You may be grieving the absence of your partner less than the fact that you were unhappy together, or the fact that you didn't put much energy into being happier, or the fact that the very day they died, you were planning to leave them.

Planning to leave. At that last session was Ali already planning to leave this pretty planet? Before we said goodbye I tried to tell her I was sorry the choir had not worked out more profitably for her, but she cut me short. 'Don't you go feeling bad about that,' she said, and even at the time I registered a sudden urgency in her voice. 'Don't you feel bad about anything at all, ever. You did everything you could. You've been brilliant.' She'd cancelled the previous week's session, for which Steve and I had paid in advance, and she insisted on refunding us. I stood back, lifting my arms in protest, but she stepped forward and forced the notes into my hand.

Ali gave so much, and found it so hard to receive. Another member had brought her garden flowers in a jam jar; a sweet, small gesture, but I could see that it was more than she could bear, and she asked me to keep them 'in case the water spilt in her car'. I poured the water away and gave her back the flowers and jar, and she took them quickly, shoving into her bag the chocolates that I had rushed out to buy. I wonder if those tokens of our affection and gratitude made it past the first rubbish bin.

You always wonder, with a suicide, what you could have done. I've been going round telling myself and everybody else who's expressed any anxiety, that I am sure there was no way we could have helped. Nothing anybody could have done. If being so musical couldn't help, how could they, or I, have found a way? But I do blame myself, if I'm honest. I do. At the same time as admiring her, delighting in her, I was always bloody terrified for her, but I just sat in the stalls and watched the precarious beauty of her voice, her whole being, smash into the barrier.

Guillermo might have said that all this self blame is

just ego, and maybe my ego is giving itself delusions of grandeur, imagining that I could drastically alter the course of somebody else's life, especially somebody who never asked me to try, indeed made it clear that she wanted nothing of the sort. This is even crazier than imagining that musical expression is a sure fire antidote for mental illness, or that religious faith is. I've always rolled my eyes when people say things like 'How could God let this to happen to me, when I've always been a good Christian?', or 'How can God be good if he allows the innocent to suffer?' I always want to say, 'Come on – if your religious position depends on a world in which no suffering occurs except to people who in your opinion deserve it, it won't have much of a shelf life. Do you not read the papers? Do you never look out of the window, or around the room? Life is full suffering, massive, unfair suffering, and religion or spirituality don't hoover it up any more than music does.'

Lots of suffering in Ali's life. Some suffering in everyone's life, including mine. Helping isn't the same as neutralising or abolishing pain. Who or what could have helped Ali? Maybe we all did help her in some way, just as her music did. For all I know, making a glorious sound herself and teaching us to enjoy our voices sustained Ali for many years, and I know that some of her time on this pretty planet was joyful, because I saw it. That glow when she tuned us up like the merry organ and stood back, like the artist she was, to survey her work; that was real. And I notice that I'm singing, under my breath, but a little more freely, a song we practised at the end of Clare's session. It was written by Ali Burns in response to the current grief and worry about climate change, but it seems right for this situation too. It goes: 'Do not carry a heavy heart; do not carry such a heavy heart. Do not bear the weight of the whole dark mountain...'

I have a plan. I'm going to keep going back to that choir, enduring the nauseous bus journey and the hanging around, and I'm going to get my voice back, and I'm going to learn that song through and through and sing it with my new choir buddies, and that will be the new song in my heart. It will help me, and I can almost imagine that at some cosmic, indescribable level, it might help Ali too. That's the plan. But on the chorus: 'You are the turning tide,' my voice breaks, and I have the strongest feeling that this will be one of my false starts.

How Now?

RODNEY, WHO I suspect has been reading the newspaper for the last few chapters, has turned up beside my desk to ask where I am, nowadays, with the medical stuff. He trusts that I am at least up to date with all my routine tests?

I scribble four words on an NHS invitation to send in a stool sample - they have optimistically included an obscene little plastic pot, as if the sight of it would override my previous carefully worded refusals - and stick it back in its official envelope, then turn to Rodney. He sits down on my old typing chair, the one that didn't support my upper back enough. Normally quite frugal, I spend vast sums on physical support.

I explain to Rodney that I don't have any of the routine tests. From time to time I inform my GP that I don't want them, and at least once I've filled in an opt-out form, but it doesn't stop the reminders coming. When, as happened this morning, a test or an appointment has actually been arranged, I scribble a refusal on the letter, return it to its envelope and put it back in the post, resenting the second class stamp. Bland denial seems to be the NHS's approach to would be opters out. It happened to a Facebook friend only last week, a woman who had been terrified by a 'false positive' last year. 'Why can't they leave me alone?' she wailed, and sympathetic responses popped up, one of them suggesting CBT for 'medical phobia'.

I took proxy exception to that. My Facebook pal does not have a phobia, which is an irrational fear of something harmless, such as house spiders or even, apparently, buttons. Spiders don't warn you that you might have a life-threatening illness, then take weeks to confirm that you haven't, then point out that you might have one by this time next year. Buttons don't push cameras on sticks down or up your orifices, tearing your sensitive tissue and causing infections or worse. Yes, Rodney, it happens. Just Google it.

I offer my keyboard, but the chair shoots away, propelled by Rodney's indignant foot.

'Look here. Suppose you've got one of these beastly tumour things, and you don't get any treatment until it's too late?'

'Suppose I've not got one of those beastly tumour things, and they do an colonoscopy, and tear my bowel, and I get septicaemia?'

'Dash it, that hardly ever happens.'

'Doesn't it? How do you know? I know two people who've ended up with a perforated bowel, just this year.'

'Burghhh…. Anecdotal so-called evidence. That's not scientific.'

'Rodney, I was told that nobody got severe lumbar puncture syndrome when I obviously had it myself. I don't trust their statistics.'

Rodney stands up to run his fingers along the bookcase, as if hoping to produce evidence for his own position, but finds only novels and poetry.

'Dammit, you can't just ignore the science. There are

studies, there's evidence. Are you saying you don't trust the doctors, or the NHS, or... or the Government?' Rodney is growing more British by the moment, but I expect his approach translates to other nationalities.

And, yes, I am saying that I don't trust them. Isn't that sad, especially with all the advances in modern medicine?

'Modern medicine!' says Rodney, giving up and striding to the window. 'Look how many people survive, who would have died, ooh, a hundred years ago.'

He must be right there. Penicillin is certainly a wonderful thing, though we have abused it for so long, over prescribing for ourselves and the whole food chain, that it is losing its efficacy, and we may soon find ourselves back to square one. But that isn't the point. Why can't Rodney grasp what I'm saying? I have another go.

'Just because some people are surviving illnesses that would have been fatal last century, doesn't mean that the modern approach is doing no harm.'

'Hang on. Are you one of those antivaxers?'

Rodney positions himself in front of my desk, licks his lips and sticks out his chest. He knows he is on safe ground here. In for the kill!

Ha! Not so fast, Rodney. My blood is up too, but I speak with benign smugness.

'Not at all. I believe that vaccination works. I'd risk making other people ill by not being vaccinated. I don't risk making other people ill by not being tested for all these cancers.'

Rodney's shoulders droop, and his foot nudges a ping pong ball abandoned under the table by a passing cat. 'Well, if you were my mum, I'd be very worried. Suppose you've got a tumour, here and now, and it's getting bigger.

You'd regret not being tested, right?' He blows his nose and looks away, as though already standing at my graveside, bemoaning my foolhardiness, but politely, as befits my newly deceased status. 'She knew her own mind, Claire did, she wouldn't be swayed.'

Would I regret it? Would I? Impossible to say, without a controlled trial in which one Me was tested, treated and recovered; another Me was tested and nothing happened; still another was tested and injured in the process, and so on.

To complete the set, we would need a Me who was tested, treated, suffered horribly from the treatment and died anyway. This is the path that I especially want to avoid. I tell Rodney that, and he winces, aiming a morose kick at the ping pong ball. An interested set of whiskers appears round the door.

'But it wasn't so bad for Mum! She got through the chemo and all, and she's fine now. Why wouldn't that happen to you?'

I think it just wouldn't. As well as the eye surgery and the lumbar puncture, I've reacted badly to the majority of pills and ointments I've ever been prescribed. Conventional medicine just doesn't seem to suit me. It sounds a bit pathetic, put like that. Pathetic, but also profoundly true.

Guillermo told me once that my voice would wobble until it came from a place of absolute truth. Here is the truth, Rodney:

Of course I would be upset if I found I was seriously ill, but I would prefer to know that the cause of my illness was my genetic makeup, or my lifestyle, or environmental factors, rather than having voluntarily submitted to medical tests which, as well as potentially causing physical harm, would stress me out and threaten the balance that I've painstakingly achieved from non-medical interventions. For me, none of the tests are worth it, and neither is much of the treatment.

There, Rodney. That is my truth.

Rodney thinks I should have the tests anyway, but he sounds a bit shaken.

'How are you doing?' I ask.

Steve steps over the cat, wheels the spare typing chair back to the desk, plops himself down on it.

'It's hard work being Rodney. I'm running out of steam, standing up to you.'

'You do look tired.'

'I'm scared. I think Rodney won't follow you down this route because he's scared. It is horrible, thinking of you with untreated cancer. Are you saying you wouldn't have any treatment, really?'

I don't like seeing him like this, his blue eyes guarded and looking off to the side.

'Well, I might when it comes down to it. Who knows?'

Sometimes I think I'd have the surgery, but draw the line at radiation. Sometimes I think I'd tolerate radiation but not chemo. Surgery, though, with its chances of waking up – oh, God! But could that be worse than voluntarily swallowing some potion, Socrates-like, knowing that in my body, the chemo drugs would behave like the poisons they are?

For some reason this talk of cancer feels academic, though that makes little sense, with one in two people getting it nowadays. If we are talking new medical conditions, rather than the ones I already have, my dread is of cataracts or glaucoma, something requiring (cue silent, internal screeching) eye surgery. That genetic thing my sister had, Fuch's Dystrophy, that makes you blind if not treated with corneal transplants. My sister came through surgery without complications and can see better than ever, but then she's a true Rodney, a much stronger Rodney than Steve is now, after decades of living with me, urging me to see the GP and then helping to deal with the fallout.

Faced with a choice of blindness or surgery myself, I'd probably opt for the knife. But some procedures are carried out without a general anaesthetic, not that they necessarily work, so you have to actually see - look at, I believe - the knife. Oh God! By avoiding my GP, I don't get offered tests or treatments for my neurological symptoms any more, but an American doctor whom I met through the Nystagmus Network swore that the null point surgery had improved no end, and suggested that even now, it would be worth having the operation again. No. No! Oh, GOD!

God makes no comment, but Steve puts a cool hand on the back of my neck and asks me what is wrong. I hint at the possibility of future eye surgery, whereupon Rodney exits stage left and Steve, the real Steve, goes quite pale, his own black pupils in his own blue eyes scuttling in horror.

That helps.

Finale

THIS IS A piece of life-writing, not an A Level essay or a set of instructions. In this final chapter I am not going to summarise my points so far, still less advise the reader how to apply them to their own life. I am a body psychotherapist, not a self-help guru. I can only suggest that we all feel our bodies, take note of our experiences, and always act with at least some reference to our guts.

I can suggest these things, not make them happen. My life would be quite different if I acted on my own understanding. In our house in Cumbria there is a dedicated yoga room with a sea view and a wood block floor, equipped with straps and blocks and other objects for making a whole gamut of postures safely possible. ('Engineer if necessary,' Drew used to say, 'And if that doesn't work, over-engineer'.) Some days I make use of this wonderful space, and of the years of expert teaching I received in London, finishing each practice more aligned and calm and pain free than when I started. Some days I do this, most days I just intend to. At least three practitioners have carefully shown me a method of walking which improves my mobility and reduces my joint pain, and there is a flat, mile long path close by, perfect for practising. So I walk there twice a day, morning and evening, right? Wrong. Twice a week if I'm lucky. The only thing I do consistently is avoid medical interventions which my gut forbids. And I'm quite good at arranging my day to allow moments of lying on the floor with my eyes closed, which is beneficial and free, and not too much trouble even for me.

I am not a science fiction writer, but still I would like to finish with a peek at those controlled trials where different versions of Me are living their different lives. I push open the door of the fantasy lab, where I'm instantly dazzled by complexity and motion, so that I screw up my eyes and cover them with my hands. It turns out that the degree of neurological damage I was born with cannot be uniquely tested for. Other variables have been introduced. In a gap between my fingers whirls a kaleidoscope of Mes, advancing and retreating, smiling and screaming, beloved and desolate. The mortal remains of a confident young Me, hit by a car after drinking cough mixture in the park, are replaced by a venerable musician who, able to read sheet music comfortably, found her vocation early. There's a cheerful child with a head posture, whose parents said no to null point surgery, laughing into the face of a mother who tilts her own head to match. Then there are other Mes, in the kaleidoscope's pitchy depths, born in war zones and refugee camps. There are scenes which make me screw tight the portholes of my eyes, which make even failed procedures in a well-intentioned hospital, followed by slow recovery in a quiet room, a very small thing to bear. How real they suddenly seem, the new characters in this tale, making their appearance on the final page! Maybe that past-life regression, which I resisted so firmly in an earlier chapter, has finally done its job.

Guillermo would have no truck with all this nonsense; he would tell me to stay in the present. 'Just drama, just stories! Get out of your own way! Feel your feet on the ground, both of them, look, if I push you, you topple. That's better. Breathe - be breathed. Remember, respiration is inspiration'. Somehow Elaine is here too; she smiles her wide white smile and steps up to lay her hand on my head, and my midline shimmers into place. Marianna stands across the circle, knees slightly bent, spine beautifully aligned, her posture a teacher in itself. Drew appears from the shadows and nudges my foot with his own, and I transfer the weight to the outsides of my soles. It seems that the whole choir has formed a circle, all the choirs I have sung with, Steve by my side, Miranda opposite, and there is Ali revolving in the middle, lighting up each face she smiles upon, raising her hands to lead us. Guillermo places his own hand between my shoulders and tells me, tells all of us, 'think of your neck – *here* - being made of white butterflies, feel their delicacy, their movement. Open your mouths, wider. Now, sing!'

Epilogue

I COMPLETED THIS book at the end of 2019 and have been preparing it for publication in March and April 2020, a time that will go down in history as the months the COVID19 pandemic established itself in the UK.

My book talks about medical interventions, sometimes with disappointment or frustration, even fury. Do my responses still seem reasonable, seen from this new perspective? Every Thursday at 8pm I join my neighbours in applauding, amongst others, the NHS staff; all of them, not just the doctors and nurses. There is no doubt that huge numbers are being heroic, in its original sense. I wonder how it must feel to be a medic or care-worker receiving this accolade who does not want to be heroic, but who wants instead to be safe, and to keep their families safe. It must be hard.

Watching their epic efforts from the relative comfort of my sea-view lock-down, I experience some of the same unease about the government's response to this crisis that I feel about my own experiences of medical interventions. Are they really taking into account the whole picture, the whole person, the whole nation? Is the understandable desire to prevent loss of life from the virus being sufficiently balanced against the potential suffering, even death, from economic collapse, from the painful isolation that may lead to excessive drinking, domestic violence and even suicide, not to mention the corrosive effects of stress and fear and lack of purpose? We were already concerned about social media contact replacing face-to-face social interaction; how is the new increased reliance on talking to 'holograms' rather than flesh-and-blood loved ones, eventually going to pan out?

I don't know the answers, obviously. These are questions for history. I can only hope that when statistics are published, and plans made for our response to the inevitable next crisis, the whole picture will be taken into account.

Acknowledgement

MUCH THANKS TO Nicola Mason without whose generous gifts of time, encouragement, advice, sympathy, humour and proof-reading you would not be reading this, and to Jim Belben for his thoughtful advice. Also to Shaun Levin for his excellent 'Write A Book In 30 Days' online workshop which produced the first draft. Also to Guillermo Rozenthula, Richenda Corcos, Elaine Gregory and everyone else who appears in it, and to Izzy Thorne and everyone else who said it was worth publishing. Thank you.

About the Author

CLAIRE ENTWISTLE GREW up in Surrey, lived most of her life in London. She now works as a Body Psychotherapist and writer from her home overlooking beautiful Morecambe Bay in Cumbria, along with her artist husband Steve, AKA Rodney, at least some of the time.